# HOPE

## THROUGH EYES OF FAITH

---

**SHRINK YOUR BODY
GROW YOUR SOUL
REFRESH YOUR SPIRIT**

---

*Idella Pearl Edwards*

All scripture, unless otherwise noted, is taken from the HOLY BIBLE, NEW INTERNATIONAL VERSION®. Copyright © 1973, 1978, 1984 by International Bible Society. Used by permission of Zondervan Publishing House. All rights reserved.

Scripture quotations marked "MSG" are taken from THE MESSAGE. Copyright © 1993, 1994, 1995, 1996, 2000, 2001, 2002. Used by permission of NavPress Publishing Group.

Scripture quotations marked "NRSV" are taken from the New Revised Standard Version Bible, copyright 1989, Division of Christian Education of the National Council of the Churches of Christ in the United States of America. Used by permission. All rights reserved.

Scripture quotations marked "NKJV" are taken from the New King James Version. Copyright © 1982 by Thomas Nelson, Inc. Used by permission. All rights reserved.

FRONT COVER PHOTO: Granddaughter, Christine Andersen
BACK COVER PHOTO: By Kathy DeYoung

© Copyright 2012 Idella Pearl Edwards. All rights reserved. No part of this publication may be reproduced or transmitted without permission.

CONTACT: info@idellapearl.com
WEBSITE: www.idellapearl.com

Printed in The United States of America.

Dedicated
to
Every man, woman and child
Who has ever struggled
With the physical limitations
And emotional stress
Of an overweight body.

My God will meet all your needs
according to his glorious riches
in Christ Jesus.

*Philippians 4:19*

# CONTENTS

| | |
|---|---|
| Forward by Rev. Ken Burgard | 1 |
| Introduction | 2 |
| Poem - The Diet | 7 |
| Eeewww, What a Mess! | 9 |
| How Much is Enough? | 11 |
| Stone Cold | 13 |
| Every Litter Bit | 15 |
| Arms of Love | 17 |
| Beatrice Page | 19 |
| Playing With Fire | 21 |
| When in Rome | 23 |
| Encased in Cement | 25 |
| Pure Poppycock | 27 |
| Wanna Dance? | 29 |
| Just for Me | 31 |
| The Big Picture | 33 |
| The Bites of Life | 35 |
| A String Attached | 37 |
| What's in Your Mouth? | 39 |
| Flip-Flops & All | 41 |
| Control Your Monsters | 43 |
| Beary Good | 45 |
| Spitting Nails | 47 |
| Surprise!! | 49 |
| I'd Rather Be Fishing | 51 |
| Secrets | 53 |
| The Key To It All | 55 |
| Cat Got Your Tongue? | 57 |
| Farmer Bob | 59 |
| Unruly | 61 |
| Stop That Train! | 63 |
| Childlike Faith | 65 |
| Mirror, Mirror | 67 |
| His Mysterious Ways | 69 |
| 2 + 2 = 4 | 71 |

| | |
|---|---|
| Take Charge | 73 |
| Stop! | 75 |
| Mine! | 77 |
| Attention! | 79 |
| The God Who Sees | 81 |
| Who's in Charge? | 83 |
| Heart's Desire | 85 |
| Make Every Effort | 87 |
| On Thin Ice | 89 |
| Dead Things | 91 |
| Freedom | 93 |
| Fight the Good Fight | 95 |
| In Perspective | 97 |
| A Positive Light | 99 |
| Throwers and Pack Rats | 101 |
| The Right Resources | 103 |
| Rejoice in Great Riches | 105 |
| Spoiled | 107 |
| The Cold Drizzles of Life | 109 |
| Getting the Axe | 111 |
| Thank Goodness | 113 |
| Going Through the Motions | 115 |
| Common Sense | 117 |
| Sweat Equity | 119 |
| I Hate Snakes | 121 |
| Too Blind to See | 123 |
| Taste and See | 125 |
| Completing the Circuit | 127 |
| Service With a Smile | 129 |
| The Defuser | 131 |
| Abundant Life | 133 |
| Life Packs a Punch | 135 |
| Frustrated | 137 |
| Welcome | 139 |
| Finish the Race | 141 |
| Hungry? | 143 |
| Ask! | 145 |
| One Man's Trash | 147 |

| | |
|---|---|
| Cover All Your Bases | 149 |
| Heart of a Servant | 151 |
| Take Refuge | 153 |
| What Did You Say? | 155 |
| A Rainbow Wannabe | 157 |
| Caught Off Guard | 159 |
| Danger! Danger! | 161 |
| Trust | 163 |
| Recipe for Disaster | 165 |
| It's All About Balance | 167 |
| Addicted to Mediocrity | 169 |
| The Gift of Freedom | 171 |
| Cut Out the Noise! | 173 |
| Crabby | 175 |
| Laughter, The Best Medicine | 177 |
| The Best Laid Plans | 179 |
| Decontamination | 181 |
| Remember Who You Are | 183 |
| Choose Life | 185 |
| Itching To Be Stitching | 187 |
| When God Says Go | 189 |
| Going Batty | 191 |
| First Impulse | 193 |
| Unconditional Love | 195 |
| Slow Fade | 197 |
| Odoriferous | 199 |
| Storms Of Life | 201 |
| Famous Last Kick | 203 |
| Leaving A Legacy | 205 |
| Dream On | 207 |
| Conclusion | 209 |
| Scriptures on Hope | 211 |
| Poem - Tempted | 212 |
| Poem - How Great? | 213 |
| Acknowledgments | 214 |
| About the Author | 215 |

# FORWARD

Idella Edwards is a blessing to our church family at Aldersgate United Methodist Church. She is a gifted encourager, for the church, the staff and the pastors (myself among them). Her work with the *Body and Soul* ministry at our church has helped many to grow closer to their Lord, to lose weight and build community while doing so.

Idella's creativity extends to poetry, songwriting and the sharing of devotions in the written word that she has prayerfully created in *"HOPE, Through Eyes of Faith."* You hold in your hands stories of her life, poems she's written and words of encouragement for you as you consider the spiritual dimensions of losing weight and becoming healthier.

May these devotions be a vehicle for the grace of God in your life. I pray you will be encouraged as you read, listening to your sister in Christ, as she shares from her experiences and brings an uplifting and, at times, challenging word to you as you walk the path toward a healthier body, soul and spirit.

In Christ,

*Rev. Ken Burgard*

(Rev. Ken Burgard is the associate pastor at Aldersgate United Methodist Church in Marion, Illinois. He is a gifted Bible teacher, working in the areas of Christian Education and Missions among other responsibilities at the church. He is a graduate of the University of Dubuque Theological Seminary.)

# INTRODUCTION

Dear Readers,

Thank you for choosing to read this book. I pray God will speak to your heart and you will receive the blessing for which you are searching. These encouragements are for the body, soul and spirit. The Apostle Paul, in his message to the church in Thessalonica, prayed for his friends – especially for the body, soul and spirit of each one. *"May God himself, the God of peace, sanctify you through and through. May your whole spirit, soul and body be kept blameless at the coming of our Lord Jesus Christ."* (1 Thessalonians 5:23) The purpose of this book is to nourish all three.

## THE BODY

Born in 1940, I have been overweight most of my adult life. I have tried every diet under the sun to lose weight, with some short-term success, but never enough to make a life-style change. I never drank alcohol, but I believe my addiction to food was just as severe. I could never eat just one cookie without eating six or eight. Once I began eating, I felt I could not stop, even when I was already miserably full. In 2007, after many years of fluctuating between 230 and 240 pounds, I joined a weight-loss group at our church (Aldersgate United Methodist Church in Marion, Illinois) called "Body and Soul." This spiritual group was started by Suzie Reis. I am grateful for her obedience to the Lord which has helped me and many others to win a victory over self.

The "Body and Soul" group encouraged abstinence from white sugar, white flour and over-processed foods. With the adoption of a balanced diet of wholesome nutritious foods, the encouragement of the group and dependence on God for the power to change, my physical and emotional bondage was gradually decreased and for the first time I felt strong enough to make wise choices with my head rather than eating from compulsion.

## THE SOUL

We are more than just a body with physical and emotional needs. God created us as spiritual beings and we are privileged to be created in His own image. *"So God created man in his own image, in the image of God he created him; male and female he created them."* (Genesis 1:27) When God created us, He planted a magnet in the depths of our souls to draw us to Himself.

Our Body and Soul group used God's word to discover how it applies to our lifestyle choices. Our theme verse was Luke 10:27: *"Love the Lord your God with all your heart and with all your soul and with all your strength and with all your mind."* Loving God with heart, soul, strength and mind is of primary importance if we want to find the true joy and satisfaction the body, soul and spirit crave. Recognizing that God is worthy to receive our total allegiance and devotion is the first step in attaining a healthy soul.

## THE SPIRIT

There is a difference of opinion among scholars as to the meaning of "our spirit" in the Bible. I believe our spirit represents our will and our desire. The Apostle Paul explains to us that the spirit works in opposition to the flesh. *"For in my inner being I delight in God's law; but I see another law at work in the members of my body, waging war against the law of my mind and making me a prisoner of the law of sin at work within my members."* (Romans 7:22-23)

The solution to the battle between body and spirit is for us to have the "mind of Christ." Philippians 2:5 tells us that our *"…attitude should be the same as that of Christ Jesus."* It is my prayer that through these meditations you will discover the blessings and rewards that come to us from a generous, loving God when our bodies, souls and spirits are in harmony with Him!

## LET'S BEGIN OUR JOURNEY TOGETHER

Each of us reading this book would love to look into the not-too-distant future and see ourselves doing a victory dance of body, soul and spirit. Before the hope of the future can become a reality however, we must look to the past.

One of the saints of the past that has influenced my life is E. Stanley Jones. Jones' life was greatly changed during a revival on the campus of Asbury College in Wilmore, Kentucky. He said the Holy Spirit liberated him from a sense of superiority.

He was considered to be the "Billy Graham" of India where he served as a missionary for over sixty years. E. Stanley Jones started a movement of spiritual retreats called the United Christian Ashram. My husband and I were on the Board of Directors for the Oklahoma United Christian Ashram for many years. In the early 1970's, we were privileged to hear Jones preach in Chillicothe, Ohio.

E. Stanley Jones has been an inspiration to thousands because, in addition to his spiritual beliefs, he put those beliefs into action by dedicating himself to the service of God - body, soul and spirit. He was a pure example of loving the Lord with heart, soul, strength and mind and his neighbor as himself. I have included some of his spirit-filled prayers in some of my devotionals.

The saints of the past can be stepping-stones to victory as we imitate their faith and faithfulness to guide our actions and attitudes. There are many saints we can admire from Bible times and throughout history.

If we look at images of the saints on stained glass windows in churches, we might say the definition of a saint is someone who lets God's light shine through. Using that definition, there are many "saints" in our present-day churches who are worthy of our admiration and who have much to teach us about selfless living.

Another saint of the past who has greatly influenced my life is my mother, Esther Edwards. (Yes, her married name is the same as my married name.) She passed away at the age of 100. For years, she played the piano for the Senior Center and even played a piano concert at her own 100$^{th}$ Birthday Party. She consistently looked for ways in which her life could be a blessing to others. She was the valedictorian of her high school class in Whitehall, Wisconsin in 1925. In her speech she talked about the River of Life: "Let us hope that each one of us will steer his boat well and that the Great River of Humanity may flow on more smoothly, with a deeper happier song, because we have become a part of it."

My mother wrote the following poem at the age of 91. It reflects her generosity of spirit and a belief that each day of her life was precious.

## TODAY

In the early morning it began,
A day that will never return again.
We fill the hours with work and play
And believe we've had a pretty good day.

But then today becomes the past,
When tomorrow comes at last.
We look back and try to recall
If we had done any good at all.

Did we help anybody along the way?
Did we say, "I love you" or think to pray?
Did we teach our children right from wrong?
Did we brighten our day as we sang a song?

Now we come to the end of another day
And tomorrow will become
Another today.

*~ Esther Edwards*

My mother spent her entire life giving to others. She was the epitome of selfless living. She lived the last 28 years of her life in our home, so I am fully aware of what she believed and that belief did not vary from what she practiced. Her life was a blessing. God desires for our lives, as well, to be a blessing to others, both physically and spiritually.

There is not one day of our lives of which we can say, "It's not that important. I always have tomorrow." Each day is a precious gift to be lived to its fullest to the glory of God. And may God help us remember the goals that are now so fresh in our minds so forgetfulness will not steal our resolve and consume our victory. Come with me as we begin a journey of body, soul and spirit that will make a difference. May your hope become reality!

*Blessings,*

*Idella*

## THE DIET

I started a diet. I know it's time!
I'm on my way to a body sublime!

But I miss my chocolate and hot buttered bread,
Instead I eat rice cakes with all-fruit spread.

Low-calorie soup, oh me, oh my!
If I eat one more bite, I think I will die.

While others are enjoying double-chocolate mousse,
I'm having celery and carrot juice.

Weighing and measuring and calorie counting,
The desire to abandon the diet is mounting.

But I'll dig in my heels, press on toward the goal,
I'll take time to pray and feed my soul.

I know I will make it for I'm not a quitter!
There's much more to life than a fried apple fritter.

Someday I'll look back at all this and say,
"You'll never guess what I USED to weigh!"

*~ Idella Pearl Edwards*

So here's what I want you to do, God helping you:
Take your everyday, ordinary life -
your sleeping, eating, going-to-work,
and walking-around life -
and place it before God as an offering.
Embracing what God does for you
is the best thing you can do for him.

*Romans 12:1 (MSG)*

## EEEWWW, WHAT A MESS!

One of my favorite memories is of our granddaughter Jackie singing a solo at age three at the Annual Talent Show in our church (Green Valley United Methodist Church in Henderson, Nevada). The song began with, "I'm bringing home a baby bumblebee. Won't my mommy be so proud of me!" The song told of the bee stinging her and how she squashed it with her hands and wiped it on her dress. The next line in the song, which Jackie performed with the great drama of a 3-year-old, was, "Eeewww, what a mess!"

I had my own mess a few weeks ago when I opened my purse to retrieve a ballpoint pen. We had been to McDonald's that day with our grandchildren, David and Christine. When cleaning up the table, I grabbed what I thought was an unopened package of caramel sauce the grandkids had not used for their apple dippers and threw it into my purse. Evidently it HAD been opened. "Eeewww, what a mess!"

Sadly, there are those of us who can look at our lives and say, "Eeewww, what a mess!" Our finances are out of control, our relationships are out of control and our eating habits are out of control.

There are consequences for messes. The little girl in Jackie's song received consequences from her mommy for soiling her pretty dress. Jackie dramatically ended her song with, "Ouch! She spanked me!"

The messes in our lives each have their own consequences. Financial messes can create severe hardships in the family. Messes in our relationships can leave us angry or depressed. Out-of-control eating habits can mess up our health and our self-esteem.

Some messes might be avoided or resolved by using a little wisdom and/or diligence. If I had thought to check the seal on the caramel sauce before I threw it into my purse, I could have avoided the goo. But I was able to clean it up with a little diligence. Some of the messes in our lives are not as easy. We may need a little help. In fact, we may need a lot of help. If our eating habits have been out of control for a long period of time, we may need the help of a support group to reprogram our faulty thinking and increase our motivation. And we definitely need God's help.

The disciples were in a mess one time when a violent storm at sea threatened to sink their boat. They called out to Jesus to save them. With a simple command, *"Peace, be still!"* (Mark 4:39) Jesus rebuked the winds and the sea and there was great calm. Although Jesus gives no guarantees that more storms will not come, we know that when we place our trust in Him and listen to His voice, He can tame the angriest waves.

Perhaps when you look at your life, you are tempted to say, *"Eeewww, what a mess!"* Ask Jesus for His help. Whether our storm is the result of circumstances or our own negligence, Jesus specializes in cleaning up messes.

> O Lord God, Father Almighty, purify the secrets of our hearts, and mercifully wash out all the stains of sin.
> ~ Galilean Sacramentary (7$^{th}$ Century)

**FOOD FOR THOUGHT**

~ Is my life in a mess? If so, how? Why?

~ What could I have done to avoid this mess?

~ Is there anything I need to do before Jesus can begin the cleansing?

# HOW MUCH IS ENOUGH?

How much is enough? How much of any one thing do we need to make us happy? If something makes us happy, will a larger amount of the same thing make us even happier? It sounds logical but it doesn't always work that way. Many of the things that bring us joy also have the capability, in excess quantities, of stealing that same joy. Even the good things in life have limits.

1) Pets are good, providing companionship and love, but it might get a little expensive to feed 18 dogs and 23 cats. 2) Medicine is good, but too much medicine could cause problems worse than the original sickness. 3) Sunshine is good, but after living for three years in the Mohave Desert, my skin cried out for a little moisture. 4) Rain is good, but after spending three years living on a river in West Virginia that flooded twice a year, I would have preferred a little less moisture. 5) A nice breeze is good, especially on a hot summer day, but after living in Tornado Alley for 14 years (also known as Oklahoma City) we would have preferred a little less wind. 6) Love is good, but if we hold hands all day it will be difficult to tie our shoelaces. 7) Food is good but too much can raise havoc with our health, our self-esteem and our relationships.

How much is enough? It's hard to imagine getting too much of a good thing, but it can happen. We lived in Oklahoma City at the time of the 1995 Murrah Federal Building bombing.

When rescue workers ran out of supplies, the need was advertised on television. Within an hour, a new announcement was made to stop sending supplies. The response had been so great that it created an overabundance, and the cars attempting delivery were lined up for blocks, hampering rescue efforts.

We accept limits in most areas of our lives, but for whatever reason, we resent having to put a limit on our food intake. Yes, food is good, but even if we choose the most nutritious of foods and do not limit our portions, the results could be disastrous. How much is enough? It may depend on whether we are trying to use food to satisfy a physical hunger or an emotional one. When we attempt to fill an emotional need by overeating, it will NEVER be enough.

If we use the proper quantity of food to satisfy our physical hunger and allow God to satisfy our emotional and spiritual hunger, the food is enough and God is enough. The life of the Apostle Paul was filled with both blessings and problems. Since his satisfaction came from God, he discovered he could be content regardless of how much he had. He said: *"I know what it is to be in need, and I know what it is to have plenty. I have learned the secret of being content in any and every situation, whether well fed or hungry, whether living in plenty or in want."* (Philippians 4:12)

"How much is enough?" When we know beyond a shadow of doubt that God is enough, our contentment will never be contingent upon a second helping.

> O Almighty God! Eternal Treasury of all good things! You fill all things with plenty. Let your Providence be my storehouse, my own necessities the measures of my desire; but never let my desires of this world be greedy, nor my labor immoderate, nor my care vexatious and distracting; but moderate, holy subordinate to your will, the measure you have appointed for me.
> ~ Jeremy Taylor (1613-1667)

FOOD FOR THOUGHT

~ How much will it take before I am satisfied?

~ Do I use food to satisfy a physical hunger or an emotional one?

~ Is God enough for me?

## STONE COLD

I love stones – not rough ordinary gray rocks, but smooth polished stones with interesting patterns and colors. Our family spent many hours on Lake Superior searching for agates. The best time to find agates is usually after a storm when the waves have churned up the rocks and tumbled them toward shore. Agates are easier to spot when they are wet so we would wade barefooted in the water and search until our feet turned blue from the cold water. We were usually rewarded for our efforts.

One Ash Wednesday at church, we were asked to pick out a stone from a large bowl. I was intrigued. I took my time, choosing an unusual and attractive stone. It was jet black, smooth to the touch and filled with variegated gray stripes. At the end of the service, we were invited to spend some time thinking about the stone each of us had chosen and what sin it represented. Then we were to place our stone into a large bowl of water representing The Sea of God's Forgiveness. By that time I was becoming attached to my pretty little stone but, because the stone represented my sin, I knew I had to give it up.

The longer we stubbornly hold on to our sin, the more attached we become. It was difficult for me to give up my own sin of an overindulgent lifestyle when, in 2007, I was at an unhealthy 240 pounds. I held that stone for many years and had become very fond of it.

Am I ever tempted to pick up the stone of a poor lifestyle again? You bet I am - especially when one of life's stressful storms churns me up and tumbles my life upside down. As our pastor, Rev. Tim Ozment, said: "That stone has no life of its own  - only the life we give it." The stone of an unhealthy lifestyle sends messages of promised satisfaction, but has no ability to deliver those promises.

Satan tempted Jesus in the wilderness, *"If you are the Son of God, tell these stones to become bread."* (Matthew 4:3) In Matthew 4:9, he also told Jesus, *"All this I will give you…if you will bow down and worship me."* We face those same temptations every day. Satan asks us to take the temporal things of this world and turn them into nourishment for the soul. The bread Satan offers is quick and easy and tastes great going down, yet it ultimately serves *his* final objectives, not ours. John 10:10 tells us he… *"comes only to steal and kill and destroy."* He wants to steal our self-esteem, kill our energy and destroy our bodies with disease but his purposes can only be fulfilled if we listen to his voice instead of God's.

Jesus has a purpose that is completely opposite. In John 10:10, Jesus tells us, *"I have come that they may have life, and have it to the full."* Jesus offers Himself as The Bread of Life. He promises true satisfaction and He always keeps His promises. There's nothing "stone cold" about that!

> You, Lord, are the portion of our inheritance and of our cup; you maintain our lot, so that we have reason to say, the lines are fallen to us in pleasant places and we have a goodly heritage. Especially we bless you for the bread of life which came down from heaven, which was given for the life of the world: Lord, evermore give us that bread and wisdom to labor less for the meat which perishes, and more for that which endures to everlasting life."
> ~ Matthew Henry (1662-1714)

**FOOD FOR THOUGHT**

~ Am I becoming attached to my sin?

~ Which sin in my life is the hardest to give up?

~ What is God's specific purpose for my life?

# EVERY LITTER BIT

I "cat-sat" a while back for my daughter and son-in-law, Rhonda and Jim, for their four cats. Bamm-Bamm, a large, gray, lazy cat, required insulin shots. He was an easy cat to care for because of his laid-back personality and friendliness. I didn't have to search all over the house for him. I just called, "Bamm-Bamm, insulin! Bamm-Bamm, kitty treat!" He would come sauntering up and wait for me to perform my task and give him a kitty treat.

I liked giving the insulin shot to Bamm-Bamm better than I liked cleaning the litter boxes. With Bamm-Bamm, Sam, Zoey and Grimmy, there was a lot of, shall we say, accumulation. I pulled my turtleneck shirt up over my nose and used the scoop to dig in and empty out. Sometimes we don't like to do the things we have to do. Although I don't like cleaning litter boxes, I also don't like the idea of the cats having to use a litter box that is not clean. The choice is clear.

We make choices every day. I may not want to do the dishes, but if I want to eat on clean dishes, I will do something about it. I may not want to eat a healthy lunch, but if I don't want layers of added fat stored on my body, then I will choose something nutritious rather than munching on donuts. The choice is clear.

Now here is an excellent question! If the right choices are so clear, why do we sometimes make the wrong ones? It may have something to do with our stubborn nature. We want to do what WE want to do. The scripture in Psalm 32:9 may be speaking to some of us: *"Do not be like the horse or the mule, which have no understanding but must be controlled by bit and bridle or they will not come to you."*

Our son, David, came to live with us at the age of eleven from a children's home in Ohio. To put it mildly, he was quite a handful. If I scolded him for eating candy before dinner and the next night I had to scold him again for eating cookies before dinner, he would be indignant, responding with, "But you told me not to eat candy before dinner. You never told me not to eat cookies." It really didn't matter what the rule was - David had a rebel spirit.

We, on occasion, are also rebels. Since our bodies are temples of the Holy Spirit, we should not be housing a rebel spirit. Our bodies are an amazing miracle created by an awesome God. The retina of the eye alone has 130,000,000 cells. Every square inch of our bodies contains more miracles than we can count. We can insist on having our own way, but our rebellion does nothing to benefit the wonderful bodies God created for us. It may be time for us to dig in and empty out "every litter bit" of the rebellious attitudes that so easily influence our decisions. This will give us a fresh opportunity to experience all the wonderful things God has for us.

> O God my Lord, my Life, I open every pore, every cell, every tissue, every artery, every vein, every bone to you. This body, in every part, is your temple - hallowed by your presence, cleansed by your purity, and taken hold of by your purposes. O body, behold your Lord.   ~ E. Stanley Jones (1884–1973)

### FOOD FOR THOUGHT

~ If the right choices are so clear, why do I sometimes make the wrong ones?

~ How much thought do I give to consequences before I make a choice?

~ What would encourage me most to empty out my rebellious attitudes?

# ARMS OF LOVE

When our son Bruce was a small baby, I didn't get much done. It was not because I was overwhelmed with the new responsibilities of motherhood, but rather that I was fascinated with this new little life. This tiny bundle, so warm and so soft, was my gift from God. I loved to sit and watch him by the hour, filled with the wonder that I was now a 21-year-old mother and this beautiful child was mine.

One glorious spring morning, I opened all the windows. The sun was streaming in on the carpet so I laid Bruce on a soft blanket in the living room. I lay beside him while he slept, just watching him breathe and studying every tiny miracle of fingers and toes. I left for a moment to get a second cup of coffee from the kitchen.

When I returned, I was horrified to see an enormous army of ants marching steadily forward across the carpet from a nearby window toward my 3-month-old child. I ran and swept him up into my arms, snuggling him close to my heart while I retrieved the vacuum cleaner from the hall closet and began frantically sucking up ants from the carpet. I was like a mama bear fiercely protecting her baby cub. I still remember the adrenaline rush and my dogged determination that I would let absolutely nothing harm this precious child whom I loved with heart and soul.

I love the story in the Bible that tells us how much Jesus longed to sweep His children up in His arms. *"O Jerusalem, Jerusalem, you who kill the prophets and stone those sent to you, how often I have longed to gather your children together, as a hen gathers her chicks under her wings, but you were not willing."* (Matthew 23:37)

The "heart and soul" kind of love mothers have for their children is a reflection of the enormous love God has for all His children. The Bible tells us *"God is love."* (1 John 4:16) I was taught in

English class as a child that the word "is" can be like an equal sign. God and love are synonymous. God loves us! He is well aware of the temptations that are marching steadily toward us like an enormous army, but He has given us a way out. "*...God is faithful; he will not let you be tempted beyond what you can bear. But when you are tempted, he will also provide a way out so that you can stand up under it.* (1 Corinthians 10:13)

Some of the ants marching our way are following a long trail of donut crumbs. They are gaining access through the open windows of apathy or greed. Oh how God longs to rescue us!

If we would only choose to say the word, He will sweep us up into His "arms of love," and hold us closely while He provides the way of escape. He replaces the ants of temptation with the deep satisfaction of His Holy presence. We serve an awesome God!

> O God, mercifully grant unto us that the fire of your love may burn up in us all things that displease you, and make us meet for your heavenly kingdom. ~ The Roman Breviary (1099)

FOOD FOR THOUGHT

~ Which window of my soul have I left open?

~ If I just "say the word," what word do I have to say?

~ When was the last time I allowed God to hold me closely in His arms of love?

# BEATRICE PAGE

One of the great privileges of my life was getting to know a very special 92-year-old woman from a retirement community in South Yarmouth, Massachusetts. Her name was Beatrice Page. In July 2003, out of the blue, I received a letter from Ms. Page, whom I had never met. During a church service held at her retirement home, a minister shared one of my published poems. Beatrice wrote to me and said, "On a recent Sunday, your poem, 'The Butterfly', was printed on the program. I flew right up with it!" Over the next two years, until her death in 2005, Beatrice and I developed a delightful "snail-mail" relationship. Throughout the correspondence, I was filled with growing admiration for this gentle, humble, fascinating soul, but it took many letters before I discovered who she really was.

Beatrice Page was the daughter of a Boston lawyer who sent her to Germany to study dance. She later performed with the celebrated dance team of Ted Shawn and Ruth St. Denis. She married Dr. Irvine H. Page, the recipient of ten honorary degrees and a number of prestigious awards. Beatrice Page was also an author. Her popular novel, The Bracelet, is now a collector's item. It is the story of an old woman on a double pilgrimage – one within a single day, the other covering a lifetime. I bought a signed copy of The Bracelet over the Internet. The book was just as intriguing as Bea's personality. The following is a quote from her book:

"This present moment – standing on this hill, on this Saturday afternoon, staring at the tips of her galoshes – was the little fissure she had made in time, splitting the long past from the brief future. Once she moved, this tiny rift in which she had secured a foothold would close up again; past and future would be rejoined, and she would slip back into the one or be driven forward into the other."[1]

I often think about Beatrice Page. How easy it would have been for Bea to feel sorry for herself! When she began writing me, she had one blind eye, arthritic fingers and had suffered a slight stroke. It would have been tempting for her to dwell on the negative and resign herself to living with only past memories. Instead of "slipping back into the past," she reached out to the future to establish a new friendship. The blessing was all mine!

Beatrice Page, although steeped in accomplishments for which she could be proud or even boastful, simply encouraged others. Her letters were filled with glowing words of admiration for my poetry. Only later did I learn she was also a poet, writing deep and profound poems far superior to any of mine. Yet she chose to see the good in others and to minimize her own accomplishments.

We can learn many things from the life of Beatrice Page. The best way to care for body, soul and spirit may be the opposite of what we think. Instead of using teeth-grinding determination to overcome our human weaknesses, our greatest source of power may come from focusing on our blessings from God. *"Praise the LORD, O my soul, and forget not all his benefits."* (Psalm 103:2)

---

Almighty God, Father of all mercies, we your unworthy servants give you humble thanks for all your goodness and loving-kindness to us and to all whom you have made. We bless you for our creation, preservation and all the blessings of this life; but above all for your immeasurable love in the redemption of the world by our Lord Jesus Christ; for the means of grace and for the hope of glory. ~ Book of Common Prayer (1549)

---

### FOOD FOR THOUGHT

~ Do I find myself reaching for the future or dwelling in the past?

~ What tempts me most to have a pity party?

~ What percent of my time do I spend seeking my own well-being and what percent the well-being of others?

# PLAYING WITH FIRE

As a child, I had a great deal of freedom. One reason for this was that in the 1940's it was a safer world in which to live and parents didn't have to hold the reins as tightly. Another reason was that my mother worked full time and could not afford a babysitter during the summer or after school. My father was an alcoholic and my mother worked long hours to put bread on the table. She depended on the neighbors to keep an eye on me.

I enjoyed my summers. It was a time to experiment and explore. When I was seven years old, my ten-year-old brother, Bobby, took me with him to play on the railroad tracks. When a train stopped, we climbed up one of those "fun" ladders on the side of a car, waited until the train started to go and then dared each other to be the last one to jump off and roll. If the conductor saw us, he yelled at us about the dangers, but we would just laugh and run away. After all, we never got hurt. How could it be dangerous?

In the fall after school, we had fun building large bonfires out of fallen leaves. My brother and his friends dared each other to run and jump over the fire. I was never that brave. Instead, my friends and I liked to "roast" potatoes by wrapping them in tinfoil, and burying them in the fire. When they were "done" we ate them voraciously and, although we thought they were delicious, they were always burnt on the outside, raw in the middle and tasted slightly like tin.

Playing on the railroad tracks and playing with fire are not wise choices for children or for any of us. We, as adults, choose unwisely to play with fire when we choose to indulge in unhealthy eating. When the fires begin to burn out of control, the results are charred health and a burnt self-esteem. Although the statistics are clear, we adopt an attitude of immunity. Surely these things won't happen to us. We feel just fine. These are things that happen to

OTHER people. When God whispers a warning to our hearts, we just smile smugly and walk away.

We may gamble for a while and win, but eventually the games of self-abuse will backfire. As an adult, I no longer play on railroad tracks or play with fire but I AM tempted to play the odds by eating unhealthy foods or unhealthy quantities, all the while daring the flames to leap my way. Although we have knowledge and experience on our side, we sometimes act like a kid in a candy store. In 1 Corinthians 13:11, the Apostle Paul said: *"When I was a child, I talked like a child, I thought like a child, I reasoned like a child. When I became a man, I put childish ways behind me."*

Playing with fire will get us into trouble. With God's help we can put out the flames of our self-seeking and begin to use our freedom wisely.

> O eternal and everlasting God, direct my thoughts, words and work. Wash away my sins in the immaculate blood of the lamb, and purge my heart by your Holy Spirit, from the dross of my natural corruption, that I may with more freedom of mind and liberty of will serve you, the everlasting God, in righteousness and holiness this day, and all the days of my life.
> ~ George Washington (1732-1799)

**FOOD FOR THOUGHT**

~ Are my fires of desire burning out of control? Am I fanning the flame?

~ How long will I be able to gamble with my health when the stakes are so high?

~ What will have to happen before I am willing to put my childish ways behind me?

# WHEN IN ROME

We've all heard the expression, "When in Rome, do as the Romans do." If we are in a place where we are unfamiliar with the customs or traditions, we must be careful not to do or say anything that could be interpreted as offensive to the local people.

That's what our daughter, Rhonda, did in 1986 when she went on a mission trip to Costa Rica. During her two months there, she made a supreme effort to follow the customs of the local people. In a letter she shared with us:

> It was quite a culture shock. The worse thing, worse than the four-inch cucarachas, worse than the hot sun and continuous sweat, worse than the cement taking layers of skin off my hands, worse than rice and beans three times a day, worse than the stomach issues we all had…is the smell by the baño (bathroom) and the smell outside our bedroom window. We have to go outside to get to the bathroom through the pigs and chickens. I'm pretty sure what we're smelling is the slaughtering. It's not all bad though…we're all in good spirits.
>
> I would patiently take a bug out of my rice and beans and keep eating. I shared my shower willingly with the spiders and cockroaches, and my bed with the fleas (flea bites are bad!) I patiently tossed and turned all night on the heat waves in time with the moo's, oink's, cluck-cluck's, cock-a-doodle-doo's, bzzz's and ruff's. But I enjoyed myself! I really did.
>
> There's a lot to appreciate. The people are super friendly and the church family loves the Lord immensely. I really am glad I came, and I'm having a wonderful and meaningful time!

Rhonda put aside her own personal comfort for what she considered to be the mission to which God had called her. What is the mission to which God has called *us*? Most of us will never be called to go on a mission trip to a foreign country. But God is calling us to represent Christ to the world in all we do and say. Obedience to God in every area of our lives is not always comfortable. We love to be comfortable. We spend our lives working hard so we can afford the comforts of life. Being comfortable, although sometimes a side benefit of hard work, should not be our main goal. Our main goal should be to please God with our actions and attitudes, whether or not we are comfortable.

"When in Costa Rica," do as the Costa Rican's do. "When in Rome," do as the Romans do. We may not be in Rome or in Costa Rica, but we are "in Christ." Our mission, should we choose to accept it, is to put aside our own personal comfort and follow the example of Jesus in body, soul and spirit. Jesus said, *"I have set you an example that you should do as I have done for you."* (John 13:15) Therefore, "when in Christ," do as Christ would do!

---

Father, sometimes I hear your law at church. I nod my head in agreement then go out and do nothing. Worship is over and I feel good about my faith. I got what I came for; I am saved and that's enough. But in my heart I know better. I am aware that my personal salvation comes at great cost to you; I must not wrap it up and hide it safely in the closet. Instead, I should wrap it around someone suffering in the cold; I should use it to feed the hungry and demonstrate your love to all. Make me a doer of the law, Father, not just a hearer   ~ Andrew Murray (1828-1917)

---

## FOOD FOR THOUGHT

~ What personal comforts is God calling me to sacrifice for the good of others?

~ How do I find things to appreciate in the midst of my own discomfort?

~ What is God calling me to do to represent Christ to the world?

## ENCASED IN CEMENT

Our daughter, Kerry, enjoys reading articles describing, "What Kids Say About Love." One day, she decided to ask her nine-year-old son, Samuel, some pointed questions about love, even though he was "anti-girls."

- What is the proper age to get married?
  Sam: "100 - cause I want to die first."
- When is it okay to kiss someone?
  Sam: "Never - just cause. But you're supposed to ask first."
- What is falling in love like?
  Sam: "Bad, like when your cat scratches you in the eye."
- Confidential opinions about love.
  Sam: "My cat is soft and my rabbit is too. So I love them because they are soft and they aren't girls."
- Surefire ways to make a person fall in love with you.
  Sam: "If they ask, I'm gonna say NO…cause a NO is a NO!"

Most nine-year-old boys have negative opinions about girls and love. They would rather have a tooth pulled than be seen with a girl! When Sam turned 16, I suspect he changed his mind regarding an opinion or two that were, at one time, "encased in cement." As we mature, or as facts are presented, we either change our minds or add more cement.

If we continue adding layers of cement, it becomes increasingly difficult to change. We may grow comfortable with our cement and settle for less or perhaps look at the thickness of the cement and become overwhelmed at the mere thought of change.

Where do we find the strength to change? God has generously given us two sources of power – His Holy Word and the Name of Jesus. *"For the word of God is living and powerful, and sharper than any two-edged sword..." (Hebrews 4:12) "...I tell you the truth, my Father will give you whatever you ask in my name. Until now you have not asked for anything in my name. Ask and you will receive, and your joy will be complete."* (John 16:23-24) Nothing works better for breaking up cement than His Name and His Word!

Many times we don't want to admit we need this power. We think we can break through all those layers of cement using our own strength and willpower which is about as effective as trying to chop a hole in a sidewalk with a plastic spoon. Even when we finally realize we need help, we still find it hard to ask. Perhaps it is because we want to be the one in control. Or perhaps we don't ask because we really don't want an answer. We prefer the status quo. When we get to the point that we are ready to ask for help, God is there!

If we discover we have immature opinions and poor attitudes "encased in cement," we are not helpless. When we pray in God's Name and use His Word, anything is possible!

---

Lord, we pray that we may live a life worthy of you and please you in every way, bearing fruit in every good work and growing in knowledge. May we be strengthened with power according to your glorious might so that we may have great endurance and patience and joyfully give you thanks!
~ based on Colossians 1:10-12

---

## FOOD FOR THOUGHT

~ In what ways do children look at things differently than adults?

~ How stubborn am I? Are my attitudes encased in cement?

~ How often do I listen to God's still small voice of wisdom?

# PURE POPPYCOCK

Our grandson, Ben, in his junior year of high school, along with his classmates, had to write a poem to be published in a book called, "Hubris, A Student Literary Journal." The word hubris means, "The excessive pride and ambition that usually leads to the downfall of a hero in classical tragedy." Ben's poem, "Understanding," was voted by his classmates as one of the best in the class saying it was an excellent and profound piece of poetry. Here is his poem:

## UNDERSTANDING
### by Ben Edwards

Mom understands when elephant takes something.
She cries through what was once the window.
The white water jumps with the whisper of the sad story.
Of magic and butterflies, Of pumpkins and stars.
Dad understands when dishwasher runs away.
He yells through what once was the light.
The white rapids roll with the singing of the mad glory.
Of war and sleeping, Of defeat and noise.

What they didn't know is that Ben used an online kid's scrabble type of website that allows the user to move letters around to make random words and sentences. There is NO deep profound meaning behind the poem. It's simply a bunch of nonsensical random statements - nothing more than pure poppycock!

I wonder how often we ascribe value to things on this earth that are nonsensical to God. We admire those with outward beauty even when they do not display a beautiful spirit on the inside. We look up to those who have accumulated great riches whether or not they have accumulated God's wisdom. We value those in high position while God values those who are willing to be servants. God tells us in Isaiah 55:8-9, *"My thoughts are not your thoughts, neither are your ways my ways...as the heavens are higher than the earth, so are my ways higher than your ways and my thoughts than your thoughts."*

When it comes to food, we have an entirely different perspective than that of God's. When we think eating a plateful of brownies as something that will solve our problems or something that will reward us for working hard all week, how nonsensical is that?

God created our taste buds. He created foods with a vast variety of wonderful textures and flavors. I am fully convinced God intended for us to enjoy food. But He also gave us wisdom. Wisdom dictates that we are not to enjoy food at the expense of our health and well-being.

We must be careful that our "excessive ambition" to enjoy food does not lead to our downfall. God longs to bring us His joy through everything He created but in the balanced ways that benefit body, soul and spirit. When we lean too heavily on the things of this world to give us joy, it is nothing more than "pure poppycock!"

> Lord, how I love your law! I meditate on it all day long. Your commands make me wiser than my enemies, for they are ever with me. How sweet are your words to my taste, sweeter than honey to my mouth! I gain understanding from your precepts; therefore I hate every wrong path. ~ based on Psalm 119:97-98,103-104

## FOOD FOR THOUGHT

~ How much do I "hate every wrong path"?

~ What makes something valuable?

~ Which of my attitudes would God label as pure poppycock?

# WANNA DANCE?

Do you like to dance? Dancing has been an important part of history, used for celebrations and entertainment even in the earliest civilizations. Dancing figures have been found etched on cave walls even from prehistoric times. Dance was a major method of passing down stories from one generation to another.

Our granddaughters, Meghan and Colleen, do Irish Step Dancing, which is a traditional dance of Ireland. Step-dancing is performed mostly on the toes, with the torso and arms kept straight and vertical. There are many different types: jigs, reels, hornpipes, treble jigs, set dances and slip jigs.

My mother's 100$^{th}$ birthday party was held at Aldersgate United Methodist Church in Marion, Illinois in 2009. Meghan and Colleen pleased the audience by performing several Irish dances. They were stunning in their fancy dresses full of elaborate embroidery. They wore perfectly curled wigs that added a bouncy, energetic look as the curls bobbed up and down with each step. Irish Step Dancing has spread throughout the world. "Riverdance," a theatrical show consisting of traditional Irish Step Dancing, began on stage years ago in Dublin, Ireland and is still inspiring audiences today.

Dancing is a great way to tone the body and develop strong muscles. Good muscle tone increases the flexibility and grace of everything we do. It's easy to spot a dancer. Whether she's walking or reaching for something, her gracefulness is noticeable right down to her fingertips.

I was thinking about the spiritual muscles that can be used to dance for God. I love Psalm 90:14 from the Message Bible: *"Surprise us with love at daybreak; then we'll skip and dance all the day long."* Does God surprise us with love at daybreak? You bet He does – without fail, every morning! He blesses us with a brand new day and a fresh new start. The mistakes and failures of yesterday can no longer hold us captive. God provides for us an extra measure of His grace and lovingly encourages us to place our faith in His wisdom and power. Each brand new day is indeed a gift from a loving God that makes our feet want to dance.

What kind of dance pleases God? Does He expect us to jump up on the tabletops at a church potluck and do a dance that says, "Look at me! I'm sooo spiritual!"? Certainly not! Instead, God wants a dance that will glorify Him - a dance that uses the spiritual muscles of obedience and humility. Just as physical dancing is a great way to develop strong muscles, our spiritual dance will develop strong spiritual muscles which will enable us to do a victory dance! When our spiritual dance develops to the point of keeping in step with the rhythm of the Spirit, it becomes a dance of grace and beauty, right down to our spiritual fingertips.

Wanna dance? God is surprising us every day with His love at daybreak. Giving back to Him the gift of obedience in every area of body, soul and spirit is the kind of dance that pleases Him most.

> Hear, O LORD, and be merciful to me; O LORD, be my help. You turned my wailing into dancing; you removed my sackcloth and clothed me with joy, that my heart may sing to you and not be silent. O LORD my God, I will give you thanks forever.
> ~ Psalm 30:10-13

## FOOD FOR THOUGHT

~ What kind of dance pleases God?

~ Does God's love make me want to dance? Why or why not?

~ How do I strengthen the spiritual muscles of obedience?

## JUST FOR ME

Loretta Crosson, my friend at church, loaned me a book entitled, "Missionary Mama." The author, Ruth Seamands (age 94), was born in Herrin, Illinois and is a personal friend of Loretta's. She now lives in Wilmore, Kentucky. The book tells of her exciting experiences as a missionary to India – from a centipede on her pillow to jungle cats in her attic and monkeys on her roof. She writes about people brought to Jesus and lives changed. I was so excited after reading the book, I wrote a letter to the author. In her gracious reply, she shared the following story:

    Jaytee and I were married when we were twenty-one. He was a redheaded preacher with a trombone. Many different times in India we went to churches and Jaytee took his trombone. He preached awhile, sang awhile and played his trombone awhile. Villagers loved him!

    Sunday, August 29, 2010, was the anniversary of his death. Six years ago my daughter Sheila and I sat with Jaytee, she on one side of his bed and I on the other. He was dying. We soothed his face and white hair, whispering our love. He died at 8:08 p.m.

    On Sunday, August 29, 2010, I had been thinking of Jaytee all day and I was sad. I always go to the Sunday afternoon service at Hahn Manor in Wesley Village and sit on the front row so I can hear and see well. That day I was near to tears.

    Just as we were beginning to sing the first song, in the door walked a strange man with a notebook, a Bible and carrying a case for some long instrument. He sat down next to me and I gasped when he hurriedly opened his case. He took out a trombone. A preacher with a trombone! On this special day, the Lord had sent me A PREACHER WITH A TROMBONE! Then he stood up to play and sing a beautiful song which

Jaytee had often sung. The words mean so much: *"I'll Never Walk Alone."* When the Lord does something to bless us, He does it up right. It just about took my breath away. Wonderful Lord! He did it just for me![2]

Our wonderful Lord is always at work. There are so many things He does "just for me." He does these things because He cares. In 1 Peter 5:7, it tells us, *"Cast all your anxiety on him because he cares for you."* God cares when we are burdened with problems and stress. He cares when we feel inadequate and helpless. He even cares when He sees us struggling with self-control. O how He cares!

In the midst of all our struggles, we long to know someone cares. Someone does! If we cast all our anxiety on Him and open the eyes of our heart, we will know beyond a shadow of a doubt that He cares because we will see all the wonderful things He does just for us. He does them "just for you" and He does them "just for me!"

> Your love, O LORD, reaches to the heavens, your faithfulness to the skies. Your righteousness is like the mighty mountains, your justice like the great deep. O LORD, you preserve both man and beast. How priceless is your unfailing love! Both high and low among men find refuge in the shadow of your wings. They feast on the abundance of your house; you give them drink from your river of delights. ~ Psalm 36:5-8

**FOOD FOR THOUGHT**

~ Does God do things "just for me"?

~ How do I know God cares about my burdens and problems?

~ When is it hardest to cast ALL my anxiety on Him?

# THE BIG PICTURE

Our grandson, Jacob, had an opportunity during college to go to Ireland on a mission trip in 2008. He shares the following:

> God provided numerous opportunities for me to show the love of God to many people in Ireland. I was privileged to talk with an Irish woman whose cousin was suffering from an addiction to drugs. I was able to encourage her and inform her of a Teen Challenge meeting at one of the local churches. God also blessed me in conversations with many teenagers and He confirmed the call He has placed in my life to work with them.
>
> Being in Ireland opened my eyes to more of the spiritual world than before, and showed me the immense importance prayer plays in our everyday lives. The trip helped me to see more of what God wants me to do and how He wants me to do it. One way I am pursuing His plan is a college minor for Inter-Cultural Studies, Mission. With this, I hope to inspire youth to work in the mission field and help evangelize the youth of the world.

Jake sees the big picture. He sees himself as part of the larger plan of God. He has a vision of the immense possibilities for mission - not just to the youth in his neighborhood, but also to the youth of the world.

In our own lives, we often have tunnel vision. Years ago, I had a fear of flying by myself. It was not the usual fear of an airplane ride, but a fear of getting lost in the airport. I tend to be a bit "directionally impaired" and I feared going down the wrong concourse, ending up in the wrong terminal at the wrong gate and eventually on the wrong plane. My husband taught me how to get the big picture. He told me to stand still and take my time to see all the signs before I went charging off down a concourse.

Instead of charging down the hallway of good intentions, we must meditate on all the signs God has given us that lead to His master plan. That plan includes more than eating, sleeping, working and playing. It includes giving Him glory in everything: *"Whether you eat or drink or whatever you do, do it all for the glory of God."* (I Corinthians 10:31)

How do we know if our lives are glorifying God? God does not call all of us to be youth workers or missionaries or pastors. What if our gift is to be a banker or an artist or a homemaker? How do we glorify God? Simply by offering God our best and by giving Him credit for our talents and abilities.

Getting "the big picture" shows us not only the big things, but includes all the small things – like signs at the airport, or according to our scripture, even what we eat and drink. It includes the panoramic view as well as the seemingly insignificant things that infiltrate our lives every day. Once we recognize "the big picture," it reveals unlimited opportunities to glorify our Heavenly Father with body, soul and spirit.

> Almighty and most merciful Father, in whom we live and move and have our being, grant, we beseech you, that Jesus our Lord, the Hope of glory, may be formed in us, in all humility, meekness, patience, contentedness and absolute surrender of our souls and bodies to your holy will and pleasure.
> ~ Simon Patrick (1626-1707)

**FOOD FOR THOUGHT**

~ Does God have a master plan for my life?

~ What is the best way to get the big picture of what God is trying to show me?

~ What opportunities did I have this week to glorify God?

# THE BITES OF LIFE

Have you ever been bitten? When I was a baby, I was bitten by a rat. My mother heard me screaming and rushed into the nursery. When she turned on the light, she saw a large rat jumping out of my crib after it had bitten the palm of my hand!

At the age of five, I was playing in a small creek near our house and saw a large turtle. I decided to take it home to show my mommy. I put my hands on either side of the shell and picked it up only to have the snapping turtle's head shoot out and bite the back of my hand before I knew what was happening. Needless to say, I dropped the turtle and ran home crying.

When our children were small, our family did a great amount of camping. Anyone who has gone camping is fully familiar with the "bites of life!" I've had my share of insect bites – chiggers, mosquitoes, black flies, horse flies and ticks. I vividly remember one camping trip in the Upper Peninsula of Michigan. The noseeums were driving us crazy. A noseeum is a biting midge. It is a bloodsucker many times smaller than a mosquito but with a bite much more painful. They are very easy to kill – just smash them with your finger. This is great, if you see one. The problem is they are so small, you "no-see-um" until you feel the bite! They were small enough to go through the screening in our camper. At night, even with the covers up to my chin, I would suddenly jump from the sharp pinprick of a noseeum biting me on the cheek and would spend the rest of the night with my head under the covers.

The "bites of life" are sometimes dangerous, sometimes physically or emotionally painful and sometimes just plain irritating, but everyone has them. No one is immune. We have the "bites" of sour relationships, job losses, financial hardships, tornados, floods, physical disabilities, illness, disease and even flat tires.

The Apostle Paul had his share of "bites" in his lifetime. He tells us in 2 Corinthians, Chapter 11, that he has been in prison, flogged, exposed to death again and again, beaten with rods, stoned, gone without sleep, gone without food and water and had been cold and naked. He actually had much more than his share of the bites of life. Did that stop him from preaching the gospel? No! He said in Philippians 3:14: *"I press on toward the goal to win the prize for which God has called me heavenward in Christ Jesus."*

When the "bites of life" come…and they will…we do not have the option to use them as a reason to whine, complain or give up. How many times have we used them as excuses for not staying on our healthy eating plan or for not exercising? God gave us an amazing resilience. We, along with the Apostle Paul, can *"press on toward the goal"* and God will be with us every step of the way.

---

Thank you, Lord, that through you, we are more than conquerors! And thank you that neither death, nor life, nor angels, nor principalities, nor powers, nor things present, nor things to come, nor height, nor depth, nor any other creature, shall ever be able to separate us from your love, which is in Christ Jesus, our Lord.
~ based on Romans 8:37-39

---

## FOOD FOR THOUGHT

~ Which bites of life have I experienced recently?

~ Which of those bites of life am I tempted to use as excuses?

~ What does it mean to be "more than a conqueror" through Christ?

# A STRING ATTACHED

Our grandson David, at age eight, loved playing computer games. Before he was allowed to play on the computer, he first had to have a piano lesson. I quickly found David's enthusiasm for piano lessons didn't quite match mine. When I would tell him it was time for his lesson, he sometimes responded, "But I don't want to." David quickly became familiar with my reply, "OK David, you don't have to if you don't want to, but there's a string attached from the piano to the computer." He soon learned what that meant - if he didn't practice piano, he would not have the privilege of playing games on the computer. So now if I say, "That's okay, David, you don't have to if you don't want to," he responds with, "I know, I know. There's a string attached. I want to." Although his computer time is limited to one hour, those strings come in mighty handy.

If we listen closely, we can hear our conscience telling us, "It's time to exercise." Our response? "But I don't want to." Guess what? We don't have to if we don't want to, but there is a string attached. There is a string that connects our exercise to a strong healthy body. If we don't want the one, we can't have the other. Carole Lewis, who is the national director of First Place 4 Health, writes in her book, <u>Stop It!</u>, "…wanting lasting change and actually achieving it are not as simple as we may think. The body wants to do what the body wants to do. Seldom do we wake up in the morning and think, 'Yippee! I get to exercise today!'"[3]

Why do we need to exercise? Exercise can do many great things for the body. It can protect us from heart disease, stroke, high blood pressure, Type II diabetes, obesity, back pain and osteoporosis. It improves our mood and helps us manage stress. It increases blood and oxygen flow to the brain thereby improving mental alertness and it reshapes our bodies, giving us a more positive feeling about ourselves.

Most of us do not exercise regularly despite the proven health benefits. It has been said that, "The only exercise some people get is jumping to conclusions, running down their friends, side-stepping responsibility and pushing their luck!" Even when we convince ourselves we must exercise, we tend to procrastinate. Some of us are planning to start an exercise program as soon as we get enough money to buy new exercise equipment...or whenever we get caught up on all our projects...or whenever we find a friend with whom to exercise. If we want a healthy, strong body, there's a string attached. It is impossible to enjoy the benefits of exercise if we never get off the couch. We must stop procrastinating and just do it! Ecclesiastes 11:4 says it well, *"Whoever watches the wind will not plant; whoever looks at the clouds will not reap."* In other words, if we wait for perfect conditions, we will never get anything done.

No, we don't have to exercise if we don't feel like it, but now that we know there is "a string attached," we may want to.

> Lord, help each of us to show diligence to the very end, in order to make our hope sure. We do not want to become lazy, but to imitate those who through faith and patience inherit what has been promised. ~ based on Hebrews 6:11-12

### FOOD FOR THOUGHT

~ In what ways is it true that I have to "use it or lose it"?

~ Why do I procrastinate on exercising?

~ What are some ways I can make exercising more fun?

## WHAT'S IN YOUR MOUTH?

My son, Bruce shares the following story:

My wife, Mary, owned and operated a licensed day care in our home for many years. With tough budgets, she liked to save money by making her own play dough. We had some yellow popcorn oil in the pantry that she thought might work well for her play dough recipe. When the play dough was done, the popcorn oil had colored the play dough so it looked just like cookie dough. The wheels began to turn in Mary's head. She knew I liked raw cookie dough, so she and Sharon, her employee, hatched a plan.

Mary hustled out to the store to buy some chocolate chips. Back home, Mary mixed the chocolate chips into the play dough, moistened the edge of the bowl and sprinkled it with flour, placed a piece of wax paper over the 'cookie dough' and placed the bowl in the fridge. All afternoon, they chuckled to themselves thinking of the poor victim (me) who would soon be home from work.

When I finally arrived home, I followed my typical routine, putting my things down and heading straight for the fridge for a snack. When I opened the door and saw the cookie dough, my eyes lit up! Not wanting to eat in front of the day care children who were still around, I grabbed a handful, hid it from sight until I was in the hallway and then threw it into my mouth.

If you are not familiar with powdered alum, an ingredient in Mary's play dough, alum immediately sucks the moisture out of the mouth and acts like the worst puckerer ever. Boy, was I surprised! The worst part was knowing I'd been had and having to listen to Mary's and Sharon's roaring laughter.

We laugh at this comical incident because Bruce had no idea what he was putting into his mouth. In reality, the joke is on us. We sometimes have no idea what we are putting into OUR mouths either. Many foods today are over-processed so they will not spoil, thereby giving them a long shelf life to increase profits. If we look closely at each food label, we will discover some with a list of additives and preservatives so lengthy it looks like the inventory of a chemical supply room.

In the daily challenge of choosing wholesome foods, we desperately need God's wisdom. *"Oh, the depth of the riches of the wisdom and knowledge of God!"* (Romans 11:33) God's wisdom is available just for the asking. *"If any of you lacks wisdom, he should ask God, who gives generously to all without finding fault, and it will be given to him."* (James 1:5)

We have an advantage over Bruce. His "cookie dough" did not come with a label listing all the ingredients. On your next trip to the grocery store, use a little wisdom and make a practice of reading labels before choosing a product. Why? So you will know "what's in YOUR mouth!"

> Set a guard over my mouth, O LORD; keep watch over the door of my lips. Let not my heart be drawn to what is evil, to take part in wicked deeds with men who are evildoers; let me not eat of their delicacies. ~ Psalm 141:3-4

## FOOD FOR THOUGHT

~ What is the difference between knowledge and wisdom?

~ How much wisdom did I use on my last trip to the grocery store?

~ How "wholesome" is my diet for "other" things such as the books I read or my choice of television programs?

# FLIP-FLOPS & ALL

In September 2000, my friend Bonnie and her daughter Ginger were in Guatemala staying at an orphanage. Ginger Teeter Hopwood tells this story:

Mom and I were riding down a highway in a pickup truck. Dave, a staff member of the orphanage, was driving, Mom was in the middle and I was sitting in the passenger seat. All of a sudden, Dave starts yelling, "Ginger, you have to get him!! There is one of our boys from the orphanage who ran away and YOU have to go get him!" (Dave is around 350 lbs.) The response in my head was…"HUH? I'm a 29 year old, 104 lb. female wearing flip-flops...I can't do this!"

Dave pulls over to the side of the road and what do I do? I jump out and start chasing this kid. We were in a farming area…lots of little hut type houses and fields. The boy sees us and takes off through the fields. As I'm chasing him, through peoples' yards and fields, through pig pens filled with pig manure (and I have flip-flops on), all I can think of is that all of these Guatemalan women in their yards and fields are going to see this scrawny little white girl, chasing one of their own, and they are going to take off after me with pitchforks.

I finally get the boy. He is crying, and I'm feeling horrible because I have a very limited Spanish vocabulary and I couldn't tell him I wasn't going to hurt him and that it would be okay.

Bonnie shared later at the orphanage that the kids were all spreading the word. "Beware of the 100 lb. blonde girl – she will get you!"

Even with all Ginger's reservations, she was able to rescue a frightened runaway child in spite of the fact… a) she had no running shoes, b) she was not much bigger than the boy, c) she feared the women would misinterpret her motives and, d) the boy himself might misunderstand what she was trying to do. Ginger made a radical decision to burst into action and leave the rest in God's hands.

God is speaking to each one of us right now. Are we listening? He is saying, "This is what HAS to be done and YOU have to do it!" Our reply? "I can't do it! What if 'this' happens? What if 'that' happens? Besides, I'm wearing flip-flops!" If we wait for optimal conditions before we take action, optimal results will be impossible.

I wonder what would happen if we would stop procrastinating and burst into action as soon as we hear God's voice? What if we buried all our excuses and started giving God an unreserved and unqualified "Yes!" In Judges 6:14 the Lord told Gideon, "*Go in the strength you have...Am I not sending you?*" While we are waiting for optimal conditions, we are missing out on a multitude of God's blessings.

We need to go in the strength we have…"flip-flops and all!"

> Help us, O Lord, to walk humbly, prayerfully, consistently on, in the dust of our pilgrimage so that men may not stumble over us and say, "They profess only; they never do anything."
> ~ Dwight L. Moody (1837 - 1899)

**FOOD FOR THOUGHT**

~ Which excuses do I tend to bury and then dig up again?

~ What things am I more likely to procrastinate on than others?

~ Am I listening? What is God telling me to do right now?

## CONTROL YOUR MONSTERS

When my daughter, Kerry, was small, she knew how to control her monsters. She says,

> When I was six years old I lived in a place that had a large number of stray dogs. Most of these dogs were not nice friendly strays. They had been living on their own for a while and had grown distrustful of people. But somehow, much to my parents dismay, this innocent, naïve child became very good at breaking down the distrust of those dogs and, one by one, each became my friend.
>
> Fast forward a few years and you'll find a nine-year-old girl now living in a new state, feeling very out of place in her strange new surroundings. As that feeling filtered into my dreams I began having recurring nightmares. In the nightmare wild monsters would surround my home threatening and scaring me. But every single time, every time I dreamt this, I would summon my courage and bravely approach the monsters. Somehow I was able to bridge the gap of misunderstanding and their aggressiveness would disappear. Suddenly my dream was no longer a nightmare but a wonderful frolic with my newfound friends.

Kerry learned how to control her monsters. Our grandchildren, David and Christine, know how to control monsters as well. They both love music and especially "The Phantom of the Opera." Their favorite song is the beginning Overture. It is their "scary music" and when played, I have to pretend to be the Phantom and chase them.

They have two methods of escape. 1) If one of them can sneak back to the music player and switch the music to a sweetly sung song called, "Think of Me," the Phantom must instantly become nice. 2) The other method is for them to hide in the hall closet. When I open the closet door, Christine comes out hobbling on a walking cane pretending to be an old woman. Then I'm supposed to ask her, "Madam, have you seen two delicious-looking children?" She denies this, throws down the cane and they both run away. They never tire of this game. (Grandma does, of course.) But they do a good job of controlling their monsters.

How well do you control YOUR monsters? We all have monsters in our lives. There are, for example, the monsters of apathy, the monsters of selfishness or pride, the monsters of quick tempers and the monsters of greed. The list is endless. A monster that is ignored tends to become more unruly than ever. Kerry controlled her monsters by creating positives out of negatives. There is no greater asset for self-control than a positive mind! David and Christine control the Phantom by a simple decision that they will be in charge. They created the rules for the game. The Phantom has nothing to say about it.

With God's help, we are the bosses of our own bodies. We have the power to control the monstrous urges that tempt us because God "...*is able to do immeasurably more than all we ask or imagine, according to his power that is at work within us.*" (Ephesians 3:20) Are you controlling YOUR monsters?

> Summon your power, O God; show me your strength as you have done before. You are awesome, O God, in your sanctuary; you give power and strength to your people. I give you praise!
> ~ based on Psalm 68:28, 35

**FOOD FOR THOUGHT**

~ Who is in charge of my life?

~ Which negatives in my life could, with God's help, be turned into positives?

~ What do I expect to happen when I pray - immeasurably more or immeasurably less?

## BEARY GOOD

My friend, JoAnne Swafford, shares the following story:

It was a cool morning for mid-July in the Upper Peninsula of Michigan - a nice day for picking raspberries. Reluctantly, all six kids, ages 6 thru 12, would grab berry pails made from 1-lb. coffee cans. Each one had a wire for a handle and a piece of twine to tie the bucket around our waist, leaving both hands free for faster picking. When we'd whine about spending our summer picking berries, my mother would remind us that in the dead of winter, while eating berry pie, we'd be glad we spent the summer working instead of playing.

Today we would be picking along the railroad tracks. A couple years before, the railroad men had cut trees to keep the railway clear, leaving the brush piled up. This is where the largest wild berries grew. Mother had her eye on that patch of berries ever since she saw the blossoms in the spring. Six kids and my mother, with her double-barreled shotgun over her shoulder, set off for a berry-pickin' day. I didn't know who Annie Oakley was but the family would tease her by calling her that. We felt safe knowing that gun was over her shoulder.

Along the tracks was an uphill grade with tall grass and thick bushes. Big red raspberries were hanging from them. Mother lined us up like a drill sergeant, spacing us a few yards from each other. We knew the ritual. We picked as far as we could to the left, then to the right, and of course in front as far as our arms could reach. And we'd better pick our space clean!

Every once in awhile, my mother would call our names and ask how we were doing. It was time for roll call, but when she got to my sister - no answer. After a few calls she spread the bushes wide and yelled, "Answer me!!!" To her shock, she looked directly into the face of a black bear standing on his hind legs, his mouth full of berries. With a growl, the bear took off down to the railroad tracks and into the woods as fast as he could go, but not before stumbling over the gun that was laying on the tracks that my mother brought with us just in case we came upon a bear.

JoAnne's story is a "beary good" example of the shocking little surprises life sends our way in the form of temptations. Satan does not send us an email warning us that we will be tempted at 4:00 p.m. on Friday afternoon. He is a master of deception, hiding in the bushes of our apathy and carelessness. Our double-barreled shotgun is Prayer and The Word of God, but we need to keep it close by.

In Proverbs 2:1, God tells us... "*store up my commands within you.*" In Proverbs 2:6-7, He reassures us that "*... the LORD gives wisdom, and from his mouth come knowledge and understanding. He holds victory in store for the upright...*" By storing it within us, it is always within our reach! God stands ready to give us victory and that is "beary good" to know!

> O LORD, I seek you with all my heart; do not let me stray from your commands. I have hidden your word in my heart that I might not sin against you. I meditate on your precepts and consider your ways. I delight in your decrees; I will not neglect your word.
> ~ Psalm 119:10-11,15-16

**FOOD FOR THOUGHT**

~ What is the best way to store up God's commands within me?

~ In what ways have I been apathetic or careless in my care of God's temple?

~ If I visualize victory, what do I see?

## SPITTING NAILS

While I was at the hospital waiting to get an MRI, I saw a surly-looking prisoner in an orange suit being led down the hallway. He was in shackles and chains and accompanied by a big burly guard, complete with gun. I won't quickly forget the look on the prisoner's face that said, "I may be subdued for now, but if I get half a chance, watch out!" My mind played the scenario. MRI's are magnetic. If the prisoner needs an MRI, they must first remove the metal restraints. I was suddenly grateful for the powerful-looking guard. His job was to protect us should the prisoner decide to suddenly vent his anger on anyone within reach.

What makes us mad? What brings us to the boiling point? What (or who) has the ability to pull our trigger and make us spit nails? We occasionally succumb to inward or outward explosions of anger for various reasons. Stop lights? Not getting invited to a party? Someone lies to us? Noisy neighbors at 3:00 am? False accusations? Unruly children? Criminals that prey on the weak? Someone puts a scratch on our new car?

Is anger wrong? The Bible tells us, "*...Do not let the sun go down while you are still angry.*" (Ephesians 4:26) On the other hand, Jesus became angry enough in the temple to overturn the tables of the money changers who were buying and selling in God's house. (Matthew 21:12) There may be times we should not get angry, but there are also times we should get angry but don't.

We should be angry with Satan. He has bossed us around far too long. He approaches us and says, "Give me your integrity. Give me your goals and dreams. Give me your wisdom. Give me your peace." At times we are tempted to give up without a fight. He is pushing us around and we are allowing it. Satan attempts to kill our self-esteem and our motivation. He especially tries to devour our faith in the Almighty God of the Universe. Let's not hand our lives over to him on a silver platter without a fight! Ephesians

6:10-11 in the Message Bible tells us, *"God is strong, and he wants you strong. So take everything the Master has set out for you, well-made weapons of the best materials. And put them to use so you will be able to stand up to everything the Devil throws your way."*

Compared to God, Satan has no power at all. We have the power through Christ! Jesus is our security guard. If we trust in Jesus, Satan's hands are tied. Satan has been portrayed as an ominous, undefeatable adversary that we don't stand a chance of overcoming. But God's power is supreme, and through God's power, we always win. *"We are more than conquerors through him who loved us!"* (Romans 8:37)

It should make us angry when Satan tries to trip us up, entice us or sabotage our efforts to be holy. It's time to go from defense to offense, fight the good fight and "spit our nails" in the right direction!

---

Praise be to you, O LORD, God of our father Israel, from everlasting to everlasting. Yours, O LORD, is the greatness and the power and the glory and the majesty and the splendor, for everything in heaven and earth is yours. Yours, O LORD, is the kingdom; you are exalted as head over all. Wealth and honor come from you; you are the ruler of all things. In your hands are strength and power to exalt and give strength to all.
~ 1 Chronicles 29:10-12

---

FOOD FOR THOUGHT

~ What makes me angry? Why?

~ Which of my dreams has Satan stolen? Am I ready for a fight?

~ How much confidence do I have in Jesus as my Security Guard?

## SURPRISE!!

Do you like surprises?  We were very successful in surprising our son and daughter-in-law one time.  Bruce and Mary were celebrating their 1$^{st}$ wedding anniversary on the first day of Family Camp at Michigamme United Methodist Institute.  They had chosen the beautiful log chapel at Michigamme the previous year for their wedding ceremony.  They invited us to come.  We made plans immediately to fly up there, but informed them we would be unable to attend.

We sent a cassette tape in advance to be played during the event. When we arrived at camp, we hid in a room adjacent to the celebration.  Unaware of our presence, they played the cassette tape for everyone to hear.  At the end of the tape, the dialog on the tape between my husband and me went something like this: "You know, this message is so impersonal." "I agree. What should we do?" "Why don't we just walk through that door?"  And we did. It was a rather emotional reunion.

Surprises are fun.  Our loving and generous God loves to surprise us as well.  My husband and I coordinated a Lay Witness Mission at Firestone Park United Methodist Church in Akron, Ohio.  The team met for prayer before the service.  It was a glorious spring morning, the windows were open, and all the birds were singing and chirping loudly.  We stood in a circle holding hands.  One of our team members, noted for his genuine, heartfelt prayers, began to lift his voice and give God praise.  He prayed, "Lord, at the sound of your voice, even the birds hush their singing!"

At that very moment, every bird abruptly stopped singing and a hush fell on each one standing there.  We knew beyond a shadow of doubt we were standing in the very presence of God.  It was a holy moment.

My friend, Kathy DeYoung, tells a similar story. She and her husband were traveling to hear their son, Dan, sing in a choir at the State Music Contest in Rossville, Illinois. Kathy said:

> On a dark and cloudy morning, my husband and I headed to the music contest. The concert room was set up with risers in front of an arched frosted window. It was early morning and the boys came into the room and stood on the risers. The choir director raised his baton and the boys started to sing the song, "Morning Has Broken." At that precise moment the sun began streaming through the large window behind the boys. What an awesome God we have to give us such a reminder of Himself on such a dark cloudy morning.

(By the way, the boys won 1$^{st}$ place.) God loves to surprise us with joy, with sublime experiences in which we have a glimpse into the eternal. *"You have made known to me the path of life; you fill me with joy in your presence, with eternal pleasures at your right hand."* (Psalm 16:11) He has planned much more for us than just a mediocre existence. If we are looking for true joy, we must take our eyes off the pleasures of this world and turn our eyes upon Jesus. Try it. You'll be joyfully surprised!

> Because your love is better than life, my lips will glorify you. I will praise you as long as I love, and in your name I will lift up my hands. ~ Psalm 63:3-4

**FOOD FOR THOUGHT**

~ How is God's love better than life?

~ Is there a difference between happiness and joy? If so, what?

~ Can I recall a time when God surprised me with joy?

# I'D RATHER BE FISHING

I have not been fishing in years but I have many fond memories. In West Virginia, we had two choices – fishing in the river behind our house to catch channel cats or fishing in the pond across the street to catch mud cats or bluegill. I was not especially fond of cleaning 20 small bluegill to get three bites of food, and since I never figured out a good way to get the muddy flavor out of the mud cats, I preferred the channel cats.

My favorite fishing memories were the times we spent smelt fishing in a stream that emptied into Lake Michigan. Smelt are like Salmon – they swim upstream in the spring to mate. They are very small fish, about six inches long, and we caught them with nets.

We never knew when the smelt would begin their "run" so we came prepared to spend the night in the woods near the stream. We made sure we had flashlights and a delicious picnic lunch. I don't know if our children loved it because they enjoyed fishing or because they got to stay up all night. Others in the area joined us making it a great social event.

We occasionally sent a child down to the stream with a flashlight to see if the smelt were "running" yet. Once the cry of affirmation rang out, usually after midnight, we all rushed to the stream with long-handled nets and large buckets to land our catches. It took no time at all to fill our buckets to the brim and overflowing.

What does all this have to do with body, soul and spirit? Many times, we spend our Christian lives with a line in the water trying to catch God's blessings. We even bait the hook with good church attendance and faithful Bible reading. But God longs to give us blessings by the bucketful. He doesn't want us to sit around and wait for Him to nibble at our bait and bless us. He wants us to experience all He has for us and the only way that will happen is if we make sure we are at the right place at the right time listening for the cry of affirmation that He loves us. Let's give it a name. It's called submission – submission to God's will for every part of our lives, including healthy living.

E. Stanley Jones, in his book, The Way, gives a list of ten steps to victory. Step #4 is: "Consent to surrender. Christ is Lord, not you. This is the crucial step. If you slur this over, then nothing will come out right. Some bow the knee to what others will say. Others bend the knee to themselves. Everybody bends the knee to something. Life is a partnership, with God as Senior Partner."[4]

Instead of sitting idly with a line in the water, "I'd rather be fishing" with a net, scooping up God's blessings in great abundance until my life overflows. *"May the God of hope fill you with all joy and peace as you trust in him, so that you may overflow with hope by the power of the Holy Spirit."* (Romans 15:13)

---

Let your love so warm our souls, O Lord, that we may gladly surrender ourselves with all we are and have unto you. Let your love fall as fire from heaven upon the altar of our hearts; teach us to guard it heedfully by continual devotion and quietness of mind, and to cherish with anxious care every spark of its holy flame with which your good Spirit would quicken us.
~ Gerhard Tersteegen (1697-1769)

---

**FOOD FOR THOUGHT**

~ Why do I settle for less than God's best?

~ Do I consider surrendering as a weakness or a strength?

~ To what or whom am I bending my knee?

# SECRETS

We still have some of the original furniture we purchased when we were married in 1960. One of those pieces is an end table. It looks like an ordinary table but it contains secrets of the heart. If you lie on the floor with your head under the table and look upward, you will discover initials, names, a child's colorful drawing of an American flag and multiple other symbols and marks. Since I am not in the habit of lying on the floor under tables, it was years before I even realized the markings were there. That means my children had great delight in secretly writing their messages over the years while their parents were clueless to their antics.

We have another table that is one of my favorites. It is not an expensive piece of furniture, yet it is a coffee table that is sturdy and just the right size. It has a storage area underneath where the grandchildren would hide when they were small. The top of the table is filled with nicks and scratches.

When we have company, my secret is safe because I made a coverlet that hides every square inch of the top. When I remove the cover for dusting, I can identify many of the scratches, including the ones created by our teen daughter (who now has a family of her own) when she came home from working at Burger King and tossed her keys onto the table. In other words, one look at that table generates past memories that create a warm flood of sweet emotions.

Although I probably would have been tempted to be grouchy had I caught any of these memory-making acts in progress, they are now a savored collection of sentimental memories. Time has a way of helping put things into perspective. There are many things, both traumatic and ordinary, that burn themselves into our memories, shaping our thoughts and attitudes for years to come.

The chips and scars of our lives can give us cause for pity parties or overindulgence. They have the potential to destroy our self-confidence and crush our dreams. It is sometimes only after the passage of time that we are able to recognize the way God's hand orchestrated each one with our best interests in mind.

We may tend to be grouchy when things don't go the way we want them to go. We may focus on the moment and miss the big picture of God's grace. But when we remind ourselves how much God loves us, we know we can trust Him to create something meaningful out of every life event. Ephesians 1:4 in the Message Bible says, *"Long before he laid down earth's foundations, he had us in mind, had settled on us as the focus of his love, to be made whole and holy by his love."*

We can trust Him because His love for us surpasses our every imagination. Romans 8:28 can help us see those chips and scars in a new way. *"We know that in all things God works for the good of those who love him, who have been called according to his purpose."* And that's no secret!

---
O Christ, my Savior and Redeemer, I am convinced that neither death nor life, neither angels nor demons, neither the present nor the future, nor any powers, neither height nor depth, nor anything else in all creation, will be able to separate me from your love.
~ based on Romans 8:35,38-39

---

### FOOD FOR THOUGHT

~ Which life events helped to shape my attitudes about food?

~ What can be done to bury my emotional scars under God's grace?

~ Am I ready to be made whole and holy?

# THE KEY TO IT ALL

One time our daughter, Karen, locked her keys in the car with the engine running. When her husband, Dave, brought the extra set of keys, she began pushing the unlock button on the remote over and over to unlock the door but it wasn't working. (The unlock button will not work if the car is running.) She was totally frustrated and confused as to how to get into the car as she continued pushing the button. Her husband (whom Karen says is the brilliant one in the family) quietly told her, "Karen, use the key."

Sometimes we become frustrated and confused as to how to make our life work. We keep pushing the world's useless buttons to make us happy. But Jesus quietly whispers to our soul.... "Use the key." What key is He talking about? He said in Matthew 16:19: *"I will give you the keys of the kingdom of heaven..."*

It's really nice when we have the keys in life we need, but it doesn't help much if we don't use them. We have all had times when we have been less than brilliant spiritually. God trusts us with the keys to life, and we either carelessly misplace them or doubt their worth.

What do keys represent? They represent "access." There are places and things that would be unavailable to us if we did not have the proper key to access them. Are there things in the Kingdom of Heaven that are valuable and worth accessing? A silly question, indeed! Let me mention three things out of many: power, hope and love.

1) Power. What does it feel like to be helpless? Some of us have had that feeling in regard to our diet. But the keys to the kingdom will give us access to the power to overcome.

2) Hope. What does it feel like to be hopeless? We live in a society where hope is becoming a rare commodity. Even some of

our young people who initially radiated positive thinking now succumb to the dark halls of doubt. When we try to "access" a new healthy lifestyle, we look to the future and see nothing but failure. We need a new hope. The keys to the kingdom will open doors to a fresh, vibrant, growing and glowing hope.

3) Love. What does it feel like to be unloved? Even if we have friends and family who love us, we may feel unloved because we don't love ourselves. We spend our days feeling guilty and unworthy because of choices we have made. The keys to the kingdom open the doors of forgiveness, mercy and grace in abundance.

The Bible tells us God's "*...divine power has given us everything we need for life and godliness through our knowledge of him...*" (2 Peter 1:3) Everything really means everything - every key we will ever need for every situation.

What key do you hold in your hand right now? What door is God waiting for you to unlock and walk through to a new life of freedom? The "key to it all" is to use the keys God gives us!

> O God, stretch me to my utmost - and that utmost means all I can be in and through you; but don't let me cry for the moon. Help me to evaluate what I can be in you, and then let me go out for that goal with all I have and with all you can give to me.
> ~ E. Stanley Jones (1884–1973)

**FOOD FOR THOUGHT**

~ Am I feeling helpless or hopeless? Why or why not?

~ Do I ever feel unloved? If so, when?

~ Which door is God waiting for me to unlock? What's waiting for me on the other side?

## CAT GOT YOUR TONGUE?

Our daughter, Rhonda, decided to bake cookies with her daughter's help. She simplified the process by making the slice-and-bake ones called "tube cookies". Four-year-old Christine called them "tube tookies". Try saying that three times! Sometimes we, as adults, have the same problem with words. We know the words we should say, but we have trouble spitting them out, like we would a tongue twister. The right words are on our tongue but when we try to say them, they come out as gibberish or might not come out at all!

Remember all the old tongue-twister favorites? - Suzie sells seashells by the seashore; Peter Piper picked a peck of pickled peppers; A big black bug bit a big black bear, but where is the big black bear that the big black bug bit; Rubber baby buggy bumpers. Then there are the tongue twisters that may not be as familiar: - A real rare whale; Eleven benevolent elephants; Cinnamon aluminum linoleum; Unique New York; Irish wristwatch. Tongue twisters really do seem to twist the tongue. Some public speakers use tongue twisters to practice their diction. Working with tongue twisters can build phonic awareness and help develop better articulation.

Not everyone is good at saying tongue twisters. Some of us could practice for years and they would still get stuck in our throats. Tongue twisters, however, are not the only words that seem to get stuck. Many times, the words "Thank you" never emerge to an audible form.

Some people may feel thankful or may demonstrate their thankfulness with some sort of gesture, but seldom utter the actual words. We've all been guilty of failing to express these words to friends and relatives, and especially to God. The simple phrase, "Thank you" becomes a tongue twister to us and rather than expressing our appreciation, we are silent.

Everything we have is from God. James 1:17 says: *"Every good gift and every perfect gift is from above, and comes down from the Father."* The sad truth may be that "Thank you" gets stuck in our throats because we don't really feel grateful. We may think that since God created us, He *owes* us His blessings, but God doesn't owe us anything.

When we try to say a tongue twister, is it really our tongue that is having a problem or is it our brain? When it comes to expressing our thanks to the Almighty God of the Universe, it's not the tongue having trouble, or even the brain, but rather the heart.

If our hearts are in the right place, the "cat" will be unable to get our tongues and prevent us from verbalizing our gratefulness to the Almighty God of the Universe. As we pour out our words of praise, we will begin to feel so blessed and so content with what we already have that our desire for wanting more than we need will disappear.

> Lord, I will sing of your great love forever; with my mouth I will make your faithfulness known through all generations. I will declare that your love stands firm forever, for you established your faithfulness in heaven itself.  ~ based on Psalm 89:1-2

**FOOD FOR THOUGHT**

~ What things do I tend to take for granted?

~ What am I most grateful for?

~ How does praising God give me power over temptation?

# FARMER BOB

In the late 1960's, my husband and I were Lay Witness Mission Coordinators for the United Methodist Church. When a church requested a Lay Witness Mission, a team of lay persons would travel to the church and conduct meetings on Friday, Saturday and Sunday, consisting mostly of witnessing and small group discussions. The team members were people from all walks of life - doctors, housewives, lawyers, janitors, factory workers, etc. When we lived in Columbus, Ohio, one of our team members was a farmer by the name of Bob. He was probably in his late 70's and managed to burn a permanent image into my memory as one of the godliest persons I've ever known.

I've never met a man who loved people as much as Bob did. You could not be around him long without feeling his great love for the God he served and for every man, woman and child in the human race. He would tell story after story of how he was able to witness to a truck driver or a homeless man on the street. He also went on mission trips to the Philippines, Africa and Japan.

He was a poet and when a poem would come to him, he would stop plowing the field, hop off of his tractor and write it down on any scrap piece of paper he could find. I remember well the image of him standing up in front of the church, during a Lay Witness Mission, sharing his story. When Farmer Bob decided to share a poem he would begin searching through the pockets of his bib overalls one by one and bring out all these crumpled pieces of paper trying to find just the one he wanted to share. This is one of his poems:

> I enjoy little talks each day with my God
> They surely do brighten this path that I trod
> It seems he puts steps when I've mountains to climb
> If you don't believe it, just try it sometime
> Oh, what a Companion to have by my side
> Now I see rainbows where dark clouds used to hide.

Farmer Bob was an inspiration to others because he spent a lifetime growing closer to the Lord. There was no part of his life off-limits to God's control. He had the wisdom to know that whatever he gave to God multiplied back to him in spiritual blessings.

There are many ways God calls us to serve others. We are to share our material resources with those in need, offer a helping hand whenever we can, lend a listening ear and share the gospel with those who need the truth. Bob did all these things, but he also did the most important thing he could ever do for others. He set an example for us to follow of a life lived in sweet fellowship with the Almighty God of the Universe.

The only way Farmer Bob was capable of loving others so completely was because he knew, beyond a shadow of a doubt, how very much God loved him. *"We love because he first loved us."* (I John 4:19)

> Lord, help me to love you with all my heart and with all my soul and with all my strength and with all my mind and my neighbor as myself. ~ based on Luke 10:27

## FOOD FOR THOUGHT

~ Are there any areas in my life that are off-limits to God's control?

~ How often do I feel inspirations from God? Is there anything I can do to encourage them?

~ In what ways could my inspirations help others?

# UNRULY

Our granddaughter, Christine, fell in love with tea parties when she was four years old. I found a great tea party set with lots of tiny ceramic dishes at a garage sale. Christine invited Grandpa, Grandma, and her brother, along with all her dollies and stuffed animals, to the party. She had an abundance of tea party rules and enjoyed adding more as time went on.

## TEA PARTY RULES

1. Hostess must wear her best attire. (Christine's choice was her Snow White dress.)
2. Hostess must serve all the guests first before serving herself.
3. No one may take a bite of food until the hostess has taken the first bite.
4. When sipping tea, one must hold the teacup handle gently with two fingers while holding the little pinkie high in the air.
5. When wiping one's mouth, one must dab gently on each corner of the mouth.
6. No one may talk with food in his or her mouth.
7. Grandpa is not allowed to slurp tea from his saucer.
8. All dollies must refrain from giggling or they must go straight to bed.
9. Each raisin must be nibbled, not gulped.
10. Graham cracker crumbs must land on the tiny plate, not on the table.

In life, we often express a disdain for too many rules and, indeed, there may be some areas where the rules have multiplied out of control. We would love to be "unruly" in the sense of being free from rules, but it would not take long for that lack of rules to give us an excuse to be "unruly" or reckless in our behavior.

We tend to look at God's rules as a bossy intent to take away our fun. God's love for His children is so deep, so pure, so strong and so uncontaminated by the world's point of view that He made every single rule for our benefit.  When He tells us not to love the world or the things of the world, it's not because He's trying to spoil our fun but rather because He has something far superior in mind.  His purpose is to give us His joy!

*"If you obey my commands, you will remain in my love, just as I have obeyed my Father's commands and remain in his love.  I have told you this so that my joy may be in you and that your joy may be complete."*  (John 15:10-11)

We will not readily embrace the will of God if we view His commands as bothersome or oppressive. Only when we understand how very much God loves us will we realize that *every* rule was made for our benefit.  Only then will we willingly obey His voice and follow His commands.  We will discover that strictly adhering to the right rules (meaning God's rules) will bring us deep satisfaction and true freedom. If we insist on being "unruly," (meaning free of God's rules) we will miss many of the wonderful blessings God has planned for us.

> My gracious, healing Father, I come to you with this body of mine. Forgive me for the sins I have committed against it and thus against you, its Creator.  Help me to work with you to make it the perfect expression of your will.  Give me insight into the laws of my body and help me to obey them when I see them.
> ~ E. Stanley Jones (1884–1973)

**FOOD FOR THOUGHT**

~ Are there any rules in life that I view as too restrictive?

~ In what ways are God's rules for my benefit?

~ Which blessings might I miss if I insist on being unruly?

## STOP THAT TRAIN!

Have you ever stopped a train? I have! And I did it with one hand. That's the honest truth! This is how it happened…

Years ago, my husband, Jack, my daughter, Kerry, and I and were on the EL platform on the south side of Chicago waiting to board a train. The train stopped, the doors opened, and we all boarded the train…all, that is, except my husband. He had been crowded from behind, and someone had lifted the wallet out of his back pocket and took off running. My husband, being a man of action, immediately began pursuing the offender.

My daughter and I, of course, were already on the train and as the train started, I began to panic. First of all, through the train window, I could see my husband pursuing the offender down a flight of stairs, and I was concerned for his safety. Secondly, I had no clue where to get off the train or how to reconnect with my husband. I made a quick decision. I immediately reached up and pulled the emergency stop cord, which brought the train to a grinding halt. The conductor was not happy! Fortunately, I had acted quickly enough before we ran out of platform for de-boarding.

As soon as we were off the train, someone handed me my husband's wallet. Evidently the man who snatched it was in cahoots with another man and had tossed the wallet to him before running away. The partner emptied the money from the wallet, threw the wallet down and took off while my husband was chasing the man he thought had the wallet.

My daughter and I quickly descended the stairs where we had last seen my husband. We found him on the other side of the gate. The criminal had escaped and my husband had no money to buy a ticket to get back in. The whole experience was certainly a memorable one.

It was also a learning experience. I am normally not a fast thinker, but I knew I did not have time to spare if I wanted to get off that train. Admittedly, it is my natural tendency to be a procrastinator, but there was no time to delay if I wanted to stop a moving train.

The train is moving! We need to stop thinking we can "enjoy" today and make up for it tomorrow. Today is the day. Let's stop that train! We all know which train I'm talking about. It's the one heading to a place we do not want to go. It is speeding down the rails of self-destruction. It is racing toward poor health, poor self-image, depression and family stress.

Since tomorrow never comes, today is the day to "stop that train!" Will you join me? There is an emergency stop cord within our reach. When the train comes grinding to a halt, it will not be because we had the power to stop it, but because the emergency cord is connected to a Greater Source of Power. *"For God did not give us a spirit of timidity, but a spirit of power, of love and of self-discipline."* (2 Timothy 1:7) Let's "stop that train!"

> O Resurrected and Living Lord, I would know You and the power of Your resurrection in every thought, every word, every attitude, every moment of the day and night. Then I will live in power and glory. ~ E. Stanley Jones (1884–1973)

### FOOD FOR THOUGHT

~ What is the current destination of my train?

~ When was the last time I was tempted to enjoy today and make up for it tomorrow?

~ How do I make sure my emergency cord is connected to a Greater Source of Power?

# CHILDLIKE FAITH

Our family believes in prayer. We pray for the pressing needs of our friends, our church, our world and we pray for one another. A few years ago, in addition to praying for immediate family concerns, we began the tradition of choosing one family member each week, from the eldest member to the smallest grandchild, for special prayer. An email is sent to the entire family, announcing the name of the "Family Member of the Week for Prayer." It also includes a scripture dedicated to that person. The selected person can then reply with specific prayer requests.

One time when our granddaughter, Colleen, was chosen, she replied back with a specific request. At the age of seven, she could have chosen any number of good prayers such as help with school or the ability to do her best in a gymnastic competition. She chose, instead, to request prayers for her teacher, Miss Nancy, who had lost her son. It was an unselfish act from a very compassionate little girl who believes in the power of prayer.

The privilege of prayer is a gift from God. Making sure those prayers fall into the "unselfish" category is important. Another important aspect of prayer is faith. Jesus talks about faith several times in early chapters of Mark. *"Why are you so afraid? Do you still have no faith?"* (4:40) *"Daughter, your faith has healed you."* (5:34) *"Don't be afraid, just believe."* (5:36) *"He was amazed at their lack of faith."* (6:6) *"Take courage! It is I. Don't be afraid."* (6:50)

What is faith? Some think if we pray hard enough and believe hard enough, it obligates God to respond favorably. If their prayer is not answered accordingly, they believe their faith was lacking. Faith cannot be reduced to a formula. Faith is an absolute trust in God that He is big enough, smart enough and cares enough to work everything out for our good if we place the problem in His hands.

In fact, there is a reason it has been labeled as "childlike" faith. Children are experts in the "trust" department. A small child will allow us to pick him up and carry him. He does not seem the least bit worried that we might drop him. He simply trusts.

Jesus loved children. Mark 10:16 tells us, *"And he (Jesus) took the children in his arms, put his hands on them and blessed them."* Jesus does not want us to be childish, but to become "childlike" in our faith. *"He called a little child and had him stand among them. Therefore, whoever humbles himself like this child is the greatest in the kingdom of heaven."* (Matthew 18:2,4)

Children are not afraid to ask for help for anything. Why are we hesitant to ask for help when we struggle to maintain proper nourishment of body, soul and spirit? Perhaps we pride ourselves too much on being self-sufficient. We use prayer as a last resort only after all other efforts have failed. How long before we are willing to admit we cannot change ourselves and, therefore, need God's help? Praying for God to help us change is by no means a "selfish" prayer. It is an essential part of becoming our best so we might serve God better. God wants to help. He is simply waiting for us to ask with childlike faith.

> O LORD, our Lord, how majestic is your name in all the earth! You have set your glory above the heavens. From the lips of children and infants you have ordained praise. ~ Psalm 8:1-2

FOOD FOR THOUGHT

~ What are my greatest fears?

~ Which problems in life am I least likely to pray about?

~ What do I want God to help me with right now?

## MIRROR, MIRROR

Many of us have a marred self-image for various reasons. One contributing factor is the message we receive daily through the media. It continuously reinforces the erroneous belief that if our bodies are not perfect we are not worthwhile. My husband's Canadian cousin, Rev. Ernie Johns, is a retired minister. He speaks of our image problems in one of his sermons, "The Eternal Atoning Love."

> The ancient Greeks told a story about the dangers of self-love. Narcissus was a beautiful young man who fell helplessly in love with his own image. Being the son of the River God, he would sit gazing at himself in the water unable to take an interest in anything else. There are two endings to the story. In one version, he turns into a flower. This is the optimistic one. In the other, he kills himself after reaching into the water to touch himself and blurring the image. He could not stand his own distorted image.
>
> The latter ending speaks to our addictions to the self where in trying to make ourselves feel better, when we find our dream world disrupted, we repeat the same actions over and over again. We imbibe too much alcohol, try an opiate drug again and again and run off to the casino to show we are a winner not a loser. Addicts die the slow death because of their marred self-image.

Rev. Johns stressed the problems created by a marred self-image. Our inability to maintain a healthy life-style is sometimes the result of our low self-image. We put ourselves down with negative words and thoughts, which lead to negative actions of self-destruction so we, too, die the slow death.

When we look into the mirror and see who we really are – a child of the Almighty God of the Universe – our desire to appreciate and care for ourselves will blossom. When we look into the mirror and remember what God said, *"Let us make man in our image, in our likeness..."* (Genesis 1:26) then we will know beyond a shadow of a doubt how valuable we are. We are *"...fearfully and wonderfully made."* (Psalm 139:14)

Saint Augustine said: "Men go abroad to admire the heights of mountains, the mighty billows of the sea, the broad tides of rivers, the compass of the ocean and the circuits of the stars, and pass themselves by." May we not pass ourselves by, but peer into our souls for a vision of our true worth and all God intends us to be. When that vision penetrates our souls, it sets us free to love ourselves – not with a self-serving love, but with a healthy respect for God's amazing creation.

What do we see when we look in a mirror? Do we see an image that has been marred by self-abuse or self-love? Or do we see what God sees? We need to ask God's mirror the same question that was asked in the story of Snow White: "Mirror, Mirror, on the wall, who's the fairest of them all?" God's immediate response will be, "All of them. I love each one as deeply as the other!"

> I thank you, High God - you're breathtaking! Body and soul, I am marvelously made! I worship in adoration - what a creation! You know me inside and out, you know every bone in my body; You know exactly how I was made, bit by bit, how I was sculpted from nothing into something.  ~ Psalm 139:14-15 (MSG)

## FOOD FOR THOUGHT

~ What do I see when I look into the mirror?

~ What events of the past helped to shape my self-image?

~ What things about myself do I truly admire?

# HIS MYSTERIOUS WAYS!

My husband and I have been receiving the Guideposts magazine for over 40 years. The first thing I always read when the magazine arrives is a section called, "His Mysterious Ways." It tells stories of how God mysteriously and unexpectedly intervened in people's lives in such a unique and wonderful way, it removed all doubt from their minds that God is a loving God and never far away.

I experienced my own "aha" moment from God. My mother passed away at the age of 100. I chose two songs for the funeral service I knew she liked – "It Is No Secret" and "God Will Take Care of You." I wasn't at ease, however, that I had included her very favorite song. Later, as I was going through some of her things, I found a paper she had written entitled, "His Mysterious Ways," which I have typed below:

> My favorite song is "God Will Take Care of You" and I think He proved it through a dream I had one night. I had just traded in my old car for another used car (a better one, I thought) because I was planning a trip. That very same night I had a dream I was driving along and I had to turn my car sharply to my right. The right front tire blew out and my car and I went over an embankment.
>
> The next morning I was worried about the tires so I took my car down to a place where they check tires and asked them to please see if my tires were good enough for a trip. They told me my right front tire was really bad and the others weren't very good. So I bought four new tires.
>
> On my trip a little while later, I was driving along and a car coming toward me was veering into my lane, coming straight at me. I turned sharply to the right and he just missed me but I had no blow-out…thanks to the dream and my new tires and God taking care of me.

God was taking care of my mother just as He always takes care of us, but there are times we feel He is far away and think we are on our own. This causes unnecessary worry and stress because we have not solidified it in our minds that God really cares. When we are stressed out, we tend to seek comfort in the pleasures of this world.

Psalm 121 tells us where our help comes from, *"I lift up my eyes to the hills - where does my help come from? My help comes from the Lord, the Maker of heaven and earth....The Lord will watch over your coming and going both now and forevermore."* (vs. 1-2, 8) We also have the promise in Hebrews 13:5, *"...God has said,* "Never will I leave you; never will I forsake you."

My mother had a personal encounter with "His Mysterious Ways." It cemented the truth of God's love in her heart and mind. When we encounter the truth, God's ways are not so mysterious after all.

> God our heavenly Father, when the thought of you wakes in our hearts, let its awakening not be like a startled bird that flies about in fear. Instead, let it be like a child waking from sleep with a heavenly smile. ~ Soren Kierkegaard (1813 - 1855)

**FOOD FOR THOUGHT**

~ When is the last time I doubted God was close by?

~ When I am stressed out, where do I search for comfort?

~ What method does God use to speak to me?

## 2 + 2 = 4

Do you like math? My husband loves math! He frequently does calculations just for fun. He is sure to inform me the percentage of red lights he encounters while running errands. When he reads a book, he keeps track daily of the percentage of pages he has read. When he was a kid, he enjoyed zeroing in on the square root of a number by trial and error multiplication. This was not assigned homework from school but rather, simply for entertainment. In grade school, he was required to memorize the multiplication tables through the 9's, but just for fun, he memorized the tables through the 13's. He is amused when he tells people he graduated in the top 95% of his class and they don't get the joke. Of course, he also graduated in the top 5%.

Once during an organ recital, I caught him counting the number of tiles on either side of the stage in a college auditorium. He made sure I knew there was an unequal number on each side. In reality, he was at the recital only because I twisted his arm to go, so he attempted to alleviate his boredom by doing math.

I am not particularly fond of math. I can do math, but I look at it as a necessary evil and would never choose to do it for the sake of enjoyment. I definitely never choose to do math in my head if I can locate a calculator.

Math is important to God. Psalm 90:12 exhorts us to number our days. *"Teach us to number our days aright, that we may gain a heart of wisdom."* What does it mean to number our days? If we number the days we have on this earth and compare it to eternity, the brevity of life becomes crystal clear. We have no time to waste.

We procrastinate on so many things. Losing weight is one of them. Our theory is to enjoy today because we will always have tomorrow. If we take a good look at the limited number of days we have on this earth, it's easy to do the math. We have only one lifetime to give something back to God for all He has done for us.

*"Teach us to number our days"* means we must make the most of each day of our lives. CAUTION: This does not mean trying to cram more into each hour. "Making the most" is all about quality, not quantity! "Making the most" may mean spending more time in prayer soaking up God's wisdom.

Math is an exact science created by God. 2 + 2 = 4. The equal sign means that each side of the equal sign has the same measure or value. The same is true with our scripture verse in Psalm 90. If we *"number our days,"* it will be EQUAL to *"a heart of wisdom."* Our part is to do the numbering. God's part is to do the math and create in us a heart of wisdom.

---

Take my life, and let it be consecrated, Lord, to Thee.
Take my moments and my days; let them flow in ceaseless praise.
Take my hands, and let them move at the impulse of Thy love.
Take my feet, and let them be swift and beautiful for Thee.
~ Frances Ridley Havergal  (1836 - 1879)

---

FOOD FOR THOUGHT

~ Is there anything I do that might be a waste of time in God's eyes?

~ What could I eliminate from my schedule that would give me more time to concentrate on quality rather than quantity?

~ How much time do I spend soaking up God's wisdom?

# TAKE CHARGE

Our granddaughter, Destiny, is a "take-charge" little girl. We live in Southern Illinois and she lives in Northern Ohio. One night, at the age of six, she told our son, David, "I'm going to go visit Grandpa and Grandma." Thinking she was just playing a game, he said, "OK, go pack your suitcase." Within a short time, she emerged from her room, bags in hand, insisting he take her to our house immediately! David had a rough time soothing that episode over.

When David's wife, Amanda, was pregnant with a little brother for Destiny, she told us, "Destiny tells me every time I go to the doctor she wants me to tell him to get the baby out, so I can bring him home. She said she would feed him and take care of him. All I have to do is hold him, so she won't drop him. My precious girl!"

Taking charge seems so simple when we are young. We just decide what we want to do and try to make it happen. As we grow up, life becomes more complicated. Many times, it's even difficult to decide what we really want. Everything appears more complex and choices seem to have more consequences no matter which direction we choose.

Problems surface when we don't want to choose. We want to have our cake and eat it too. "Hmmm…do I want a healthy body or do I want to enjoy a second helping of lasagna?" But choose we must.

If we will admit it, none of us is completely satisfied with our current level of success. There is always room for improvement and although we know the consequences of indecision could be devastating, we tend to procrastinate.

It's time to take charge! Maybe we fail to take action because we know taking charge also means accepting full responsibility. We cannot play the blame game. We cannot make excuses. Or perhaps we are lazy and want someone else to do it. Every action needs a leader, and if we care about the outcome, it might as well be us.

Good leaders have the following attributes. 1) A good leader is a visionary. Our granddaughter, Destiny, is definitely a visionary. She has no trouble visualizing all the possibilities. 2) A good leader is passionate. Is Destiny passionate? No question there! 3) A good leader is faithful until the job is done. They do not give up easily. Did Destiny give up easily when told she could not go to Grandpa and Grandma's house right now? Our son, David, can verify she did not!

Perhaps we can learn a lesson from a six-year-old who loves to take charge. 1) Visualize the goal. What needs to change? 2) Be passionate. If the goal is worthwhile, there is no room for apathy. 3) Be faithful. Don't stop until we reach the finish line. It's time to take charge and, *"Whatever you do, work at it with all your heart, as working for the Lord, not for men."* (Colossians 3:23)

> O Lord of my life, take away from me the spirit of laziness, faint-heartedness, lust for power and idle talk. Instead grant me, your servant, the spirit of purity, humility, patience and love. Yes, O Lord and King! Grant me to see my own sins and faults and not to judge my neighbor, for you are truly blessed forever.
> ~ Saint Ephrem of Syria (4th Century)

**FOOD FOR THOUGHT**

~ Do I know what I want? Is it the same thing God wants?

~ What is my goal? If I reach it, will I battle pride? If I don't reach it, will I battle self-contempt?

~ What prize is waiting for me at the finish line?

# STOP!

CRASH!! My husband and I were seated in the living room when we heard the noise. We raced out the front door to see what happened. Our daughter, Karen, had crashed her car into the garage door. As she turned into the driveway, she noticed that our daughter, Kerry had left a pail of water in the middle of the driveway after washing our car. So Karen opened her car window and focused her attention on the pail in an attempt to miss it. She didn't notice how close she was to the garage door until it was too late.

Most of us are prone to believe it would never have happened if WE were at the wheel of the car. Let me point out that we do exactly the same thing in our spiritual lives. We are going through life on our merry way when, all of a sudden, "CRASH!" – life hits us squarely between the eyes. We didn't see it coming because our attention was in the wrong place. We tend to focus on the trivial to the exclusion of the significant. We focus on the bad instead of the good. We focus on self instead of others. We focus on the imitation instead of the real thing.

In the 13$^{th}$ chapter of Matthew, a story is told of a merchant in search of fine pearls. He found a rare pearl of great value and did not hesitate to do whatever was necessary to buy it. How did he recognize the pearl's value? Evaluation was not made with a passing glance.

The pearl merchant had probably spent a lifetime studying the qualities of fine pearls. The more one concentrates on the qualities of the real thing, the easier it is to spot an imitation!

We miss a lot of "pearls" in our lives because we are not focusing on what is true and genuine. Sometimes we are blinded by the intensity of our own desires. Many times our pathway is camouflaged by the image of past failures or obscured by the fog of self-pity. The pearls are there and we will find them if we focus in the right direction.

There are a multitude of "buckets" in the road of life to distract us. If we are sidetracked on a "bucketful of pleasure," for instance, we may be headed for an abrupt crash of our health. It's time to bring our spiritual eyes into focus and sort out what is really important so we can apply the brakes in time. In other words, it's time to "STOP!" Stop the bad habits that ruin our bodies. Stop the negative mindset that damages our emotional health. Stop the deception that stunts our spiritual growth.

Yes, it's time to STOP! Stop focusing in the wrong direction and take the advice the Apostle Paul gave to the church at Philippi, *"So let's keep focused on that goal, those of us who want everything God has for us. If any of you have something else in mind, something less than total commitment, God will clear your blurred vision - you'll see it yet!"* (Philippians 3:15 - MSG)

> O God, my Light, I looked for you in the sky. You are there, but I see you are here too, in the very nature of things. Help me to walk with your green light. Forgive me that I have walked against your red lights. I thought I was only hurting you. I was hurting myself, too. ~ E. Stanley Jones (1884–1973)

## FOOD FOR THOUGHT

~ What bucketful of pleasure is grabbing my attention?

~ How do I hurt myself when I walk against God's red lights?

~ What will help me stay focused on the goal?

# MINE!

Our Women's Society at church asked me to read a poem about daughters at a Mother-Daughter Banquet. I held our daughter, Kerry, who was not quite two years old, in my arms while reading. Kerry had two phrases that had recently become her trademarks. One was "What's that?" The other was "Mine!"

As I read the poem, she consistently interrupted me with one of her famous phrases. She pointed to the microphone and said, "What's that?" I ignored her for a while, but soon decided it might be best to answer her, and then continue reading the poem. (The audience was thoroughly enjoying my dilemma.) The next time she asked, "What's that?" I stopped reading and said, "Microphone." She responded emphatically with a loud, firm, "NO! MINE-crophone!" The audience erupted in applause, apparently enjoying her antics much more than the poem I was reading.

Through the eyes of a developing two-year-old, ownership becomes an important commodity to the exclusion of all others. Such young children have not yet learned to think of the needs of others and how to share with them. There are adults who have this same warped sense of ownership about many things. Sometimes that possessiveness pertains to food. Some have been known to hide food from their family so they could secretly eat it later when they were alone. They may spend family grocery money at a fast food drive-up, privately devouring a greasy cheeseburger and fries in the car before going home. They may even sneak candy from their children. I once read a story where a mother confessed, "It was years before my children knew that chocolate Easter Bunnies came with ears."

I had a friend who was well known for her obsession with food. Everyone knew if you wanted to talk with my friend, it had to be done before the food was served. Once the food was there, it was impossible to get her attention. She had a problem with her "fooditude," which is a word I coined to represent our attitude toward food. My friend's entire focus for the next twenty minutes was on the flavor, the texture and the appealing nature of food to the exclusion of the rest of us. I find myself doing the same thing at times, forgetting to pass food at the table or spacing out on friendly conversation while concentrating only on my taste buds.

We all have a tendency, at times, to yell, "Mine!" Whether it is regarding our favorite coffee cup or a particular pew at church, we clutch it symbolically to our chest. We also cling to the "fooditude" that we have a right to use food any way we please to satisfy the desires of the moment. The Bible explains that everything belongs to God. *"The earth is the Lord's, and everything in it, the world, and all who live in it; for he founded it upon the seas and established it upon the waters."* (Psalm 24:1, 2)

God has given us the task of being stewards. We are called to be good stewards of our time, our resources, our relationships and yes, even good stewards of everything that goes into our mouths. Nothing is "mine." It is all HIS!

> Lord, give us weak eyes for things, which are of no account, and clear eyes for all your truth. ~ Soren Kierkegaard (1813-1855)

## FOOD FOR THOUGHT

~ What is my fooditude?

~ In what area of my life am I the best steward?

~ Although everything belongs to God, are there some things I have labeled "mine"?

# ATTENTION!

Our son, Bruce, tells the following story about our grandson, Brad.

    When Brad was 10 years old and playing for his soccer club, he was one of the bigger kids so his coach was having him do all the throw-ins from the sidelines. It had been raining all week so the soccer fields were very sloppy with standing water in some places.

    Suddenly sometime early in the second half, we noticed Brad was handing off the throw-in duties to another player. Then we noticed after Brad would clear the ball by kicking it down to the other end of the field to our offense, he would uncurl his fingers and gently look inside his hand. We finally got his attention from the sidelines and shouted, "What do you have in your hand?" To which he mouthed the word, "frog." Brad played almost the entire second half of the match with a tiny frog in his hand.

I'm sure Brad's coach would not have approved. He would have preferred that Brad's full focus be on winning the game. Brad is now an excellent athlete and does his best to give full attention to every moment of the game, but his attention and admiration for that moment in time rested fully on one of God's tiny living creatures. Only God can make a frog, and no one appreciates that quite so much as a ten-year-old boy!

It's important to focus on winning the game. But I'm wondering if sometimes it's okay to deviate from all our rules and regulations and appreciate what's right in front of us.

Maybe it's alright to leave the dust on the furniture and help our child catch a butterfly. Maybe it's okay to be late for our meeting while we help a stranded motorist change a flat tire. Maybe it's time to stop and smell the roses. Since the majority of us reading this are not 10-year-old boys, we would probably prefer smelling roses to catching a frog. But the real question might be…are we paying attention to what God puts right under our noses?

We have a tendency to charge through each day with a planned agenda so that at the end of the day, we can cross things off our list. God is speaking to us. Are we listening? He puts people and circumstances directly in our path so we might be the instruments for fulfilling His purposes. God has a plan for our lives. He wants us to be at our best physically, mentally, emotionally and spiritually. In fact, He wants us to be holy. *"But just as he who called you is holy, so be holy in all you do, for it is written, 'Be holy, because I am holy.'"* (I Peter 1:15-16)

What's getting your "attention?" Whatever it is, does it fulfill God's purposes? God may not expect us to stop and pick up a frog today, but if we pay attention, He may be telling us in His still small voice to pause and appreciate the small wonders He places directly under our noses.

> Blessed be your glorious name, Lord, and may it be exalted above all blessing and praise. You alone are the LORD. You made the heavens, even the highest heavens, and all their starry host, the earth and all that is on it, the seas and all that is in them. You give life to everything, and the multitudes of heaven worship you.
> ~ based on Nehemiah 9:5-6

**FOOD FOR THOUGHT**

~ When was the last time I stopped to smell the roses?

~ Am I willing to put my agenda aside to fulfill God's agenda?

~ Since I'm human, how can God expect me to be holy?

# THE GOD WHO SEES

While living in Las Vegas, Nevada, we met some extremely nice people. If I had a choice, however, Las Vegas would not have been my selection for a hometown. It might be a fun city to visit, but we are not gamblers and did not enjoy living there.

One thing we did enjoy was an abundance of out-of-town guests ... relatives and friends who had never been to Las Vegas and now had double reason to go there. They could finally get to see all the sparkling lights and perhaps even catch a glimpse of a movie star or two. While they were in our home, we could catch up on each other's lives and renew our friendship.

One unique aspect of living in Las Vegas was the frequent sound of police helicopters flying over our house. Most homes, ours included, have a backyard swimming pool with high cement block privacy walls. The walls made a great hiding place for those who broke the law. The police would frequently shine the bright searchlight of the helicopter into each yard in search of criminals on the run. It seemed to us that the crime rate in Las Vegas was higher than most places we had lived. Every time our backyard exploded with light, we knew it was possible a crime had been committed.

In Genesis, Chapter 16, Hagar fled from Abraham's wife, Sarah, and hid. God found her. Hagar said, *"You are the God who sees me."* (vs. 13) Yes, God is the God who sees each one of us, but He doesn't need a helicopter or a searchlight.

In the Garden of Eden, even though Adam and Eve tried to hide from God, He saw them and knew what they had done. He sees us as well. There are many times I have tried to hide from God, either by ignoring Him or by busying myself in mundane tasks, thinking He will not notice, but God always sees my heart and my motives.

There is a vast difference between the police helicopters with their searchlights and the warm floodlight of God that penetrates our souls. Both have a goal to protect. The police are protecting innocent citizens by apprehending criminals whereas God is trying to protect us from ourselves, even when we are not so innocent. He knows we can be our own worst enemy.

When we make the choice to sabotage our bodies with excess quantities of food, He sees. His searchlight exposes our self-centeredness and greed. Yet God demonstrates His great love for us in a very tangible way just as He did for Adam and Eve. Even after they disobeyed Him, He bent down and made clothing for them from the skins of animals. (Gen. 3:21)

Yes, we are prone to disobedience and yes, God is the God who sees. Yet He bends down to bless us. He offers His protection as He shines the light of His love into our hearts so we might discover the pathway to His blessings.

> O Lord our God, most mighty and merciful Father, I your unworthy servant, do once more approach your presence. Let the bright beams of your light so shine into my heart, and enlighten my mind in understanding your blessed word, that I may be enabled to perform Your will in all things, and effectually resist all temptations of the world, the flesh and the devil.
> ~ George Washington (1732-1799)

### FOOD FOR THOUGHT

~ Is there anything I'd like to keep in a dark corner away from God's light?

~ Why would God need to protect me from myself?

~ If God floods His light on the pathway to His blessings, why do I sometimes prefer to walk in the dark?

# WHO'S IN CHARGE?

Our grandson, Joseph, in Oklahoma City, wrote a story when he was in early grade school. This is his story exactly as he wrote it – with the exception of a few spelling corrections.

### SUPER JOE SAVES THE DAY

An alligator ate a person that was 40 years old. He was a dad of many children and teenagers. They got eaten by the alligator. Someone has to do something. It's Super Joey! "You stop it, alligator!" Then he struck back! He missed and then he did his super blast! Then the alligator dodged the blast but the blast followed the alligator everywhere he goes. Super Joe liked to see the alligator blown to smithereens. And the alligator did! And Super Joe saved the day again. The end.

Why do kids like superheroes? Even adults like the image of a superhero. Who among us is not disgusted with criminals that prey on the weak, stealing purses from little old ladies and abducting young children? These happenings make us feel helpless and vulnerable. We would all love to have super powers to right the wrongs of the world. We would like to be in charge. But I wonder…if we had all those powers, could we be trusted? Would we always make the right decisions? Probably not! We all know Someone who can. God is the One who is in charge.

My husband wrote a devotional entitled, "Who's In Charge Anyway?" In his devotional, he presented a few questions to ponder.

1) If we evolved from monkeys some 100 million years ago, what about the monkeys still on earth? Are they the rejects? Who's in charge anyway? 2) Is it an accident our lakes and oceans are full of water that our bodies require…water instead of, maybe, turpentine? Who's in charge anyway? 3) Our bodies can tolerate a certain range of temperature. Is it just by

chance that this is the temperature range in which we live? Who's in charge anyway?

His point was that there is Someone in charge! Our world is not an accident. We are not accidents. Everything was created on purpose for a purpose. The Bible says, *"He's God, our God, in charge of the whole earth."* (Psalm 105:7 - MSG)

How does the knowledge that God is in control impact our lives? Experts tell us that a large percentage of the irrational, impulsive and less-than-wise choices we make are stress related. Among other things, stress affects our self-confidence, our concentration is impaired, creativity is reduced, and we fail to understand the long-term consequences of decisions.

Getting rid of the stress is a matter of placing our trust in the One who is in charge. We do not need a superhero. We have a Supernatural Hero. His name is God and He's in charge!

> Holy Spirit, I see what I need; I need you. I need you, not as an occasional visitor with me, but as my constant Guest within me.
> This three-storied house of my body, mind, and soul is yours. Take over charge. Put light and heat in every room, and let the light shine from every window - with no part dark.
> ~ E. Stanley Jones (1884–1973)

## FOOD FOR THOUGHT

~ Who's in charge of my life?

~ Which of my choices invite more stress into my life?

~ Do I really believe God is on my side?

## HEART'S DESIRE

When our grandson David was six years old, he was having difficulty complying with his mother's wishes during a particular shopping trip. Rhonda repeatedly told him not to pick up and handle all the merchandise, but in typical "little boy" fashion, David could not resist picking up everything he thought was interesting. After reminding him several times not to touch things, Mommy finally told him to keep his hands in his pockets until he was out of the store and in the car.

David complied for a short time and then managed to "accidentally" knock something off a shelf onto the floor, using his elbow. He then squatted down, with his hands still in his pockets, and picked up the object by squeezing his pocket lining material around it. Did he obey Mommy's rules? Yes, in a literal sense, he did. He kept his hands in his pockets the whole time, but he was not obedient to what he knew Mommy really wanted. Although he made some effort to obey the rules, the true desire of David's heart dictated his actions.

Rules and regulations are not usually the controlling factors when pitted against determined self-indulgence. Given enough time, self-indulgence will win every time. We can be ever so determined to follow the rules, but the desires of the heart will eventually surface.

In Bible times, the Pharisees had an abundance of rules. They took great pride in how well they followed their manmade rules and condemned those who didn't live up to their standards. Jesus tried to tell them they were missing the things of greater importance – a higher rule full of love and mercy. *"You blind guides! You strain out a gnat but swallow a camel. Woe to you, teachers of the law and Pharisees, you hypocrites! You clean the outside of the cup and dish, but inside they are full of greed and self-indulgence.*

*Blind Pharisee! First clean the inside of the cup and dish, and then the outside also will be clean."* (Matthew 23:24-26)

We, too, get bogged down with the outside and neglect the inside. We take great pains to structure our lives to accomplish the most in the least amount of time. We dot our I's and cross our T's and take pride in our accomplishments. We are straining out the gnats and swallowing the camels. We are neglecting the most important thing of all – our heart. We are too busy to spend time in God's presence, too apathetic to care about our spiritual growth, too proud to humble ourselves and ask God for His help, too selfish to care how our actions affect others and too exhausted with all our busyness to sit and learn at His feet.

When we make it a priority to clean the inside of the cup, our hearts will change and we will discover that the outside is no longer the most important. When our "heart's desire" is to please our Heavenly Father, we will not be tempted to wrap our hands around things that are not God's will for our lives.

> O Lord my God. Teach my heart this day where and how to find you. Let me seek you in my desire; let me desire you in my seeking. Let me find you by loving you; let me love you when I find you. ~ St Anselm of Canterbury (1033-1109)

**FOOD FOR THOUGHT**

~ In what ways do I follow the rules to the letter but disobey God in my heart?

~ Which things do I wrap my hands around that are not part of God's will?

~ How strong a cleanser do I need for the inside of my cup?

# MAKE EVERY EFFORT

When we moved to Tornado, West Virginia, we bought a house on the Coal River. The first week we were there, my husband was sent to Green Springs, Ohio on a business project leaving me to adjust to the new house and the new community. There was a heavy downpour for three solid days and the river began to rise. I felt fairly safe because our home was a good 30 feet above the river with a large sea wall. The river was rising at a rate of three feet per hour so that night I set my alarm clock to ring every hour so I could get up and go outside with a flashlight to check on the level of the river. Fortunately, it came to within a few steps of our basement door and then began to recede.

Our river flooded a couple times a year but never reached the house. During one flood, our son, Bruce, had an idea. As he stood by the edge of the river, he could see all the "goodies" float by that the swirling waters of the river had washed from the backyards of houses upstream. He watched valuable, desirable objects float past him just out of his reach, so he decided to put forth a little extra effort to design a retrieval system. He tied a rope on a laundry basket and tossed it into the swiftly moving flood waters to haul in his treasures. Before long, Bruce had a wonderful collection of basketballs and other floatables. He even retrieved a doll for his younger sister.

When we look at our lives, many times it seems as though a river is rushing past, washing our goals out of reach. We want a healthy body. We want to look nice. We want strength and agility. We see all the wonderful things passing us by, but we have convinced ourselves that they are impossible to reach. Or perhaps we feel they are not worth the extra effort it takes to obtain them. It may depend on how badly we want them. Do we want these things enough to make the extra effort required to retrieve them after Satan has managed to swirl them swiftly away?

If our goals are the ones God planned for us, they are not impossible to reach and they are worth every bit of the effort it takes to achieve them. In fact, the Bible tells us to "make every effort!" "...*He has given us his very great and precious promises, so that through them you may participate in the divine nature and escape the corruption in the world caused by evil desires. For this very reason, <u>make every effort</u> to add to your faith goodness; and to goodness, knowledge; and to knowledge, self-control; and to self-control, perseverance; and to perseverance, godliness; and to godliness, brotherly kindness; and to brotherly kindness, love."* (2 Peter 1:4-7)

The rivers of life are not always easy to deal with, but the Bible makes it plain that a "minimal" effort to achieve the things God has set before us is not enough. We are to "make every effort."

---

Oh, Great Spirit, whose voice I hear in the winds, and whose breath gives life to all the world, hear me, I am small and weak, I need your strength and wisdom. I seek strength, not to be greater than my brother, but to fight my greatest enemy - myself. Make me always ready to come to you with clean hands and straight eyes. So when life fades, as the fading sunset, my Spirit may come to you without shame.  ~ Native American Prayer
    (Translated by Lakota Sioux Chief Yellow Lark in 1887)

---

**FOOD FOR THOUGHT**

~ What does it mean to participate in the divine nature?

~ How much effort does it take to lead a Godly life?

~ In what areas of my life do I tend to give my best effort?

## ON THIN ICE

My husband had a wonderful childhood growing up in the Upper Peninsula of Michigan in the small town of Newberry. As long as his chores were done, he had freedom to go wherever he pleased. He could play baseball in the field with his friends or go for a ride on his horse, Scout. In the winter, he would sometimes go deep into the woods on snowshoes all by himself with a Boy Scout hatchet hanging from his belt and his ice skates slung over his shoulder to go ice-skating on a remote pond.

The pond was about 1-½ miles into the woods and had a spring at one end, which meant one side of the pond was never completely frozen. Being a north woodsman at heart, he knew to check the thickness of the ice with his Boy Scout hatchet before he ventured out to skate. He was always very careful to skate only at the far end where the ice was at least six inches thick. He stayed away from the area where the ice became thin and gradually disappeared near the spring. If he had been careless or rebellious, his fun could have ended quickly in great tragedy.

When we wander too far from God's known will for our lives, we are also heading toward "thin ice." It doesn't matter whether our wandering is caused by being careless or rebellious, the danger is very real. How do we know when we are straying from God's will? Sometimes it's not difficult. When we find our thoughts and attitudes centered on what we want instead of what God wants, it might be a clue. When we find ourselves focusing on our own pleasures rather than pleasing God, we can be pretty sure we are drifting away from the solid foundation.

What does the word "wander" mean? It means to roam or stray without a definite purpose or objective. But the real question is why…why do we wander away from the known safety and security of God's will? I suspect one of the biggest reasons we wander is that we have allowed ourselves to become discontent with all our wonderful blessings and our minds imagine something more exciting and more satisfying somewhere other than where we are. We want the freedom to skate wherever we please in the great pond of life with no one telling us what to do.

The Bible instructs us to *"Make level paths for your feet and take only ways that are firm. Do not swerve to the right or the left; keep your foot from evil."* (Proverbs 4:26) It doesn't make sense to skate on the wrong side of the pond. Using our freedoms to indulge our desires and wander from truth and safety doesn't make sense either. It's a foolish thing to do. Proverbs 17:24 says, *"A discerning man keeps wisdom in view, but a fool's eyes wander to the ends of the earth."*

If we find ourselves on "thin ice," it's time to turn around and head for the solid foundation of God's love.

> O merciful Jesus, grant to me your grace, that it may be with me, and labor with me, and persevere with me even to the end. Grant me always to desire and to will that which is to you most acceptable. Let your will be mine, and let my will ever follow yours, and agree perfectly with it.
> ~ Thomas a'Kempis (1380-1471)

**FOOD FOR THOUGHT**

~ Am I skating on the wrong side of life's pond?

~ How do I know if I am straying from God's will?

~ Do I consider myself foolish or wise or somewhere in between?

## DEAD THINGS

In the 1960's we owned and operated a small motel in the Upper Peninsula of Michigan. The office of our motel in Newberry, Michigan was actually a sectioned-off part of our living room. The divider between the living room and the office was floor to ceiling bookshelves (open to both sides) with a large fish tank on the living room side, which was also easily visible in the office. We had several beautifully marked goldfish, one of which was especially large.

One night some fishermen came to the office to register for a room. They joked that the largest goldfish would make excellent bait for their hooks. The next morning, after the fishermen checked out, we noticed the large goldfish was missing. We were outraged. How could they do that! We complained for two or three days, and then one day, we noticed a smell coming from the living room. We followed our noses and found the dead goldfish. It had managed to jump out of the water and land behind the fish tank. We felt so guilty that we had blamed the fishermen for taking it.

Judging by the smell, there was no doubt our goldfish was dead. Some things appear dead but are really not. In the 5$^{th}$ chapter of Mark, Jesus went to a house where everyone was crying and wailing loudly because they thought Jairus' 12-year-old daughter was dead. He told them, *"The child is not dead but asleep."* (vs. 39) They began to laugh at Him, but He took the girl by the hand and told her to get up. Immediately, she stood up and walked around.

How about our aspirations and our dreams? Are they dead? Or are they only sleeping? We have spent our lives hoping and dreaming that we will someday be able to stop carrying around the excess weight that burdens us down. The dream seems illusive –

impossible – dead. We sometimes even laugh at the possibility that the dream could be ours.

At times it appears our dreams have been dead so long, they have begun to have a bad smell. In the story of the death and raising of Lazarus in John 11, Jesus told them to take the stone away from the tomb. But Lazarus' sister, Martha, said, *"But Lord, by this time there is a bad odor, for he has been there four days."* (vs. 39) Jesus response was, *"Did I not tell you that if you believed, you would see the glory of God?"* (vs. 40)

Some of the "dead things" in our lives are not dead, but only sleeping…waiting for us to have faith in the One who specializes in the impossible. Even if they are truly dead, God has the power to resurrect them. In Mark 9:22-23, the father of a young man who was possessed by an evil spirit came to Jesus and said, *"But if you can do anything, take pity on us and help us."* Jesus' response? *"'If you can?' said Jesus. 'Everything is possible for him who believes.'"* If we believe, God stands ready to revive our dreams that we might *"see the glory of God!"*

> I know you have plans for me, Lord, plans to prosper me and not to harm me, plans to give me a hope and a future. Give me faith to believe that all things are possible with you.
> ~ based on Jeremiah 29:11 & Mark 9:23

**FOOD FOR THOUGHT**

~ Are there any of my dreams that seem illusive? Dead?

~ Is my faith in "faith" or is my faith in God?

~ If I am able to accomplish my dream, will it bring God glory?

## FREEDOM

A few years ago I was at a large mall with my husband, my 15 year-old granddaughter and two grandsons, ages 8 and 10. Jackie and I had to finish some school shopping so we left Sam and Joe with Grandpa. When we came back, we were troubled to see Grandpa sitting on a bench alone. When we asked him where the boys were, Grandpa, (who tends to be slightly on the permissive side), said he let them play on the escalator.

Just then we looked up to see a security guard coming our way, with two grandsons in tow. It seems they were having fun racing in and out of shoppers and the security guard was afraid they would knock someone down. Sam and Joe abused their "freedom" and ended up not being free at all.

Do you like to be free? Freedom is wonderful. But it is also an awesome responsibility! It is easy to mishandle freedom. I find the more freedom I have, the more likely I will mishandle it. When I have a totally free day I seem to squander much of the time I could have used for wonderfully creative things. At the end of the day, I'm not even sure where all my time went.

Can you imagine a large city with no traffic lights where everyone is free to drive anywhere they pleased? That type of freedom would end in bondage. Seeking freedom from God's rules also ends in bondage. Sometimes, from our human point of view, it seems as though He is trying to take away all our fun. But He alone knows what is best for us and He loves us so much that every rule He gives us is for our benefit. He also gives us the freedom to choose whether or not we are going to live by those rules.

In the realm of food and nutrition, it would be easier if we did not have so much freedom. If God would only post a daily note on our refrigerator telling us what to eat and how much to eat, it would simplify things. Instead He allows us to make choices using the brain He gave us. Our brain weighs about four pounds and has 100 billion nerve cells that control our movements, our thoughts and even our emotions. God created our brains with the capacity to make wise and wonderful decisions that can benefit the miraculous bodies He gave us. But He never hog-ties us and forces us to choose wisely.

If we choose to ignore God's commands and go our own way, it may temporarily feel like freedom, but we are not really free at all. In John 8:34 Jesus said, *"...I tell you the truth, everyone who sins is a slave to sin."* Slavery is the opposite of freedom.

True freedom comes only through submission to the will of God. We will be free of the tyranny of self and free to be all that God wants us to be because *"...if the Son sets you free, you will be free indeed."* (John 8:34)

> You called me, Lord, to be free. Let me stand firm and not allow myself to be burdened again by a yoke of slavery. Help me not to use my freedom to indulge the sinful nature, but to serve others in love. ~ based on Galatians 5:1,13

**FOOD FOR THOUGHT**

~ Have any of my freedoms ended in bondage?

~ How can freedom come through submission?

~ When does freedom involve responsibility?

# FIGHT THE GOOD FIGHT

When I was young, I was never a fighter. I would run home at the mere hint of a scrabble. Besides being a big chicken, I considered fighting to be wrong. After we had our first child, I tried to teach our son, Bruce, not to fight. I also told him, "And don't EVER hit a girl." One day I noticed bruises on our son's back. I discovered that the girl next door (age 6) would chase Bruce (age 5) and pound his back with her fists as he was running away. I immediately talked with her mother and she talked with her daughter, but the poundings continued. As a young protective mother, I did a quick reorganization of my philosophies. I said, "OK, Bruce, hit her just one time. Then she will stop picking on you." As it turned out, he hit her once, giving her a bloody nose. The poundings did stop but her mother didn't speak to me for weeks.

We all need to raise our fists from time to time, not at our neighbors, but at the enemy of our souls – Satan. Our enemy makes us feel victimized, powerless and ashamed when we cannot control our own selfish behavior. So instead of fighting, we give in. This is especially true in the area of the appetite. Satan has a knack for making us feel so discouraged that we abandon all hope of change.

We should not be surprised that Satan chooses to attack us in this area. There are stories throughout the Bible regarding major battles involving food. Eve, in the Garden of Eden, saw that the fruit of the forbidden tree was pleasing to the eye, so she ate and gave some to her husband. When Esau was famished, he sold his birthright for a bowl of stew. Daniel and his friends were offered the best food in the kingdom, but vowed not to defile themselves with the royal food and wine. Jesus, after fasting for 40 days in the wilderness, was tempted by Satan to turn a stone into bread but he reminded Satan that man does not live by bread alone. In these stories, some passed the test and some did not. Food can be a delightful and essential gift from the Father who gives us all good things or food can become a stronghold of the enemy.

God gives us everything we need to be victorious. We can *"put on the full armor of God"* and take our stand against the devil's schemes. (Ephesians 6:11) He provides us with weapons of divine power. *"For though we live in the world, we do not wage war as the world does. The weapons we fight with are not the weapons of the world. On the contrary, they have divine power to demolish strongholds."* (2 Corinthians 10:3,4)

The strongholds of our lives can be demolished. We may not win every battle, but with God's help, we will eventually win the war. Then we can say, with the Apostle Paul, *"I have fought the good fight, I have finished the race, I have kept the faith."* (2 Timothy 4:7)

> Be not far from me, O God; come quickly, O my God, to help me. But as for me, I will always have hope; I will praise you more and more. ~ Psalm 71:12, 14

## FOOD FOR THOUGHT

~ Why does Satan use food to tempt me?

~ What can I do to strengthen my spiritual muscles?

~ How hard do I have to fight before I can call it a "good" fight?

# IN PERSPECTIVE

Our granddaughter Christine had an operation to repair a hernia at the age of six. Big brother, David, was feeling a little left out with all the attention she was getting. Our son-in-law, Jim, shares the following story…

> Last night, as David was probably venting frustration over Christine having received extra attention for her recent hernia surgery, he said he wanted a different sister – a sister he could play with. He wanted a sister who didn't have to worry about keeping a healing incision safe, so she could play harder. Quickly Christine sternly defended herself, saying: "David, there's more to life than just surgery! There's a whole lot of stuff. Surgery is just ONE MINUTE out of everything! There's a lot of stuff in this world, David, and surgery is just ONE MINUTE!"
>
> (Jim continues) Boy, what a wonderful video it would have made, complete with hand, facial gestures and a whole lot of love! Such a joy it was to see Christine put everything, and I mean "everything," in perspective by illustrating that even her own operation is only a very small part of life's big picture. What a joyous illustration of wisdom she portrayed!

When our daughter, Kerry, was about the same age, we took her to a drama presentation called, "J.B." depicting the biblical story of Job. Since she was unfamiliar with the story, we explained it to her before we went. On the way home I questioned her, "Did you understand the moral of the story?" Her reply was, "Of course! It means that if God gave Christians all the good stuff, then people would become Christians just to get the good stuff!" Kerry, although a small child, was able to put it all in perspective.

We, as adults, pride ourselves on our intelligence, yet we sometimes forget to put things "in perspective." Since we have an accumulation of knowledge and experience, it should be easy, but for some reason it's not. We tend to get sidetracked and to make things complicated. Putting things in perspective might mean going back to the basics, zeroing in on the necessities of life. It may mean prioritizing life to put our need list ahead of our want list. What do we really need to make us happy?

An excellent way to put things "in perspective" is to put first things first. God gives us a wonderful plan to follow. *"So do not worry, saying, 'What shall we eat?' or 'What shall we drink?' or 'What shall we wear?' For the pagans run after all these things, and your heavenly Father knows that you need them. But seek first his kingdom and his righteousness, and all these things will be given to you as well."* (Matthew 6:31-33)

We will quickly discover that if we "*run after all these things*," they will not lead us where we really want to go. Only by seeking first God's kingdom and His righteousness, will we truly be able to put things "in perspective!"

> O my Father, I have taken discipline from too many things. I have obeyed this and that. Result, I have become this and that - and nothing. But now the needle of my life, oscillating in many wrong directions, comes at last to rest in you and your Kingdom. It shall be first and always.  ~ E. Stanley Jones (1884–1973)

**FOOD FOR THOUGHT**

~ Are my needs or my wants at the top of my list?

~ How much wisdom can be found in my actions?

~ How does God's perspective differ from mine?

# A POSITIVE LIGHT

Our daughter, Kerry, who works for Dell in Oklahoma City, took a business trip to Redmond, Washington. On the shuttle one morning, she met a man named Marc who was a CIO (Chief Information Officer) of a large company. When she and her friend, Heidi, went to breakfast the next morning, she saw a couple empty seats at Marc's table and joined him, not realizing it was a whole table full of CIOs. Kerry shares the following:

> Wow! What a day we had! Heidi and I spent the ENTIRE day with these CIOs just soaking up every word they said. It was the most incredible day ever!!! They were so appreciative of us taking the time to actually listen to them and what they had to say. Heidi and I are in complete awe of what we experienced today. I never would have ever expected to end up sitting with men like this, learning from them.

As I thought about Kerry's attitude, it made me wonder how much in awe we are of spending time in the presence of God. Do we "actually listen" to what God is saying to us? Do we "soak up" every word?

Kerry went on to say, "Who wouldn't sit there and GLEAN anything and everything from them?" I like the use of the word, "glean." Gleaners are very careful not to miss anything. Nothing is wasted. To glean is to gather every last bit that is available, not just the big and obvious stuff. God wants us to glean in his fields of Bible study, prayer and meditation.

The next day Kerry and Heidi joined a different table to collaborate on some sales scenarios. Kerry said, "We took everything the CIOs fed us and led the table in designing it and then presented it to the group. Each of those CIOs came over and told us that they were blown away by our presentation because we listened and actually got what they were saying." I wonder if God would be blown away if and when we actually "get it" and start putting His teaching into practice.

Finally, Kerry told me she was proud they "were able to represent Dell in a positive light." How often do we represent God in a positive light? We are God's representation in this world. Our lives should represent the very character of God in all we do – God's love, His goodness, His truthfulness, His faithfulness, His compassion and His wisdom. We may be the only Bible some people read. Do our lives reflect all we have gleaned from Him? Do our lives reflect the image of God?

Our lives are like a candle in the darkness to those who don't know God - a candle that brings a ray of hope to those who are depressed, discouraged, confused and lost. It is not only an opportunity, but a privilege to shine. The Bible tells us to... *"Let your light so shine before men, that they may see your good works, and glorify your Father which is in heaven."* (Matthew 5:16). This is truly a "positive light."

> Bestow your light upon us, O Lord, so that, being rid of the darkness of our hearts, we may attain unto the true light.
> ~ Sarum Breviary, (A.D. 1085)

**FOOD FOR THOUGHT**

~ Do I represent God in a positive light?

~ How much time do I spend gleaning anything and everything from Jesus?

~ What areas of my Christian life shine the most?

# THROWERS AND PACK RATS

My husband is a thrower. I am a pack rat. My mother lived with us for 28 years. She was also a thrower. Other than Christmas decorations, they believed if you haven't used it for six months, it's time to throw it out.

I, on the other hand, am a saver. If there is the remotest chance that I will need in it in the next five years, I want to keep it. I have a beautiful full-length down coat in my closet that I love. I have had it for approximately 20 years. Most of those 20 years, it was too small for me but I kept thinking I might lose weight and be able to wear it. I did lose weight. But now I am living in Southern Illinois which means most of the winter days are not cold enough to warrant a full-length down coat. I want to keep it on the small chance that I may need it three or four days a year.

Although I consider myself to have the tendencies of a pack rat, I do not think of myself as a compulsive hoarder. I do not save things that are hazardous or unsanitary and the things I save do not interfere with my basic activities or create an extremely messy environment.

Both throwers and pack rats can learn from each other. (It seems God delights in combining two opposite personalities in marriage.) A pack rat tends to be the cautious, sentimental type, while throwers enjoy simplifying life so they are not encumbered with unnecessary burdens. Rev. Paul Leaming, a preacher friend of ours, said, "Whatever you own quickly owns you. If you own it, you have to dust it, repair it, store it, and in general, keep track of it." That's true. But it's also true that there are times things are thrown away that we really need and wish we had not tossed.

There are always decisions to make about throwing and keeping.

THROW: It's probably good to get rid of the food in our homes that become constant temptations to an unhealthy lifestyle. It's also a good idea to get rid of our "big" clothes. We should not save the clothes in our closet that are a size too big on the chance we may gain our weight back. We should give them away in the faith that God will continue to give us victory. It's also good to throw out our self-condemnation, our self-doubt and our self-betrayal.

SAVE: We need to save our faith and our spiritual values in a sturdy keepsake container, ready for easy access. We may sail through many days in a row with enough faith to spare, but there will come a time when we have to dig down to our toenails to find an ounce of faith to get us through. The Bible tells us, *"...do not throw away your confidence, which has a great reward."* (Hebrews 10:35)

Whether we tend to be a "thrower" or a "pack rat," each individual decision is a matter of a little common sense and a whole lot of Godly wisdom.

> Lord, help me to turn my ear to wisdom and apply my heart to understanding. I will look for it as for silver and search for it as for hidden treasure. Then I will understand what is right and just and fair - every good path, for wisdom will enter my heart and knowledge will be pleasant to my soul.
> ~ based on Proverbs 2:2,4,9-10

**FOOD FOR THOUGHT**

~ Am I a thrower or a pack rat?

~ Are there things I struggle to keep that should be thrown away?

~ In what ways could knowledge be "pleasant to my soul?"

## THE RIGHT RESOURCES

During the 1980's, we lived in Downers Grove, Illinois. My husband's job afforded him many opportunities to travel to exciting places like Bangladesh, Egypt, Switzerland, Greece, Ireland, Iraq, Kuwait, Qatar, Tanzania and many others. Jack would be gone three to four weeks at a time so it was necessary for me to handle the finances at home. He was normally the bill-payer of the family. Before he left on a trip, he would go over the bills with me and when his paycheck came in the mail, I would deposit it and pay the bills.

One time I grabbed a deposit slip not realizing it was for the savings account rather than the checking account. I deposited the money and proceeded to dutifully mail all the checks. You can guess the rest. In reality, only one check bounced. It just happened to be the check for the church, which was embarrassing to say the least.

Putting money in one account and trying to pay it out of another is not the wisest thing to do. We do the same in our spiritual life on occasion. If all our time and energy goes into the secular world and we attempt to draw on our spiritual account during a crisis, we will find it empty. It's important to build up our spiritual bank account by spending time in prayer and Bible study. We have many excuses for not doing so and the number one excuse is usually lack of time. If we suddenly had lots of time (due to an illness or a vacation, etc.) we probably would not share much of it with God. It is more likely we would find ourselves reading an entertaining novel, playing on the computer, watching television or chatting on the phone with a friend.

We can extend our sympathy to young mothers who never seem to have time to drink a cup of coffee before it gets cold and with others who, of necessity, work two or three jobs to cover financial needs. All of us need to build up our spiritual bank account and if we ask Him, God will provide the time and the means for doing so.

Bible study will greatly increase the value of our spiritual bank account. It is God's lamp to our feet and light to our path in this sinful world. It's exquisite beauty, deep wisdom and sublime truths have no equal. *"Every part of Scripture is God-breathed and useful one way or another - showing us truth, exposing our rebellion, correcting our mistakes, training us to live God's way."* (2 Timothy 3:16 - MSG)

Prayer builds up our spiritual account as well. John Wesley realized the value of prayer. He said, *"I have so much to do that I spend several hours in prayer before I am able to do it."* The Bible tells us, *"Devote yourselves to prayer, being watchful and thankful."* (Colossians 4:2) John Wesley devoted himself to prayer with an attitude of submission building up his spiritual bank account and making sure the "right resources" were available.

---

Lord, I am no longer my own but yours. Put me to what you will. Put me to doing, put me to suffering. Let me be employed for you or laid aside for you, exalted for you or brought low for you. Let me be full or let me be empty. Let me have all things or let me have nothing. I freely and wholeheartedly yield all things to your disposal. And now glorious and blessed Father, Son and Holy Spirit, you are mine and I am yours. So be it. ~ John Wesley

---

**FOOD FOR THOUGHT**

~ If I suddenly had an abundance of time, how would I use it?

~ What is the best way to make regular deposits in my spiritual bank account?

~ Is my spiritual ATM card in working order? Do I remember the password?

# REJOICE IN GREAT RICHES

Our daughter, Rhonda, was expecting a pay raise. When she received her paycheck and looked at the amount, she was astounded to find it much larger than she expected. For a moment, she was ecstatic; until common sense told her it had to be a mistake. Whoever entered the raise into the computer transposed the numbers and instead of receiving a 15% raise, Rhonda received a 51% raise. Of course she had to return the excess money.

Money tends to make us happy. There is so much we can do with money. The Funny Home Videos television show frequently shows a person receiving a fake winning lottery ticket for $10,000. Before they realize it is only a joke, they run around the room, screaming and dancing and laughing at their good fortune.

As a child, I had a recurring dream. I would climb over a tall chain link fence and on the other side I would dig a hole. After digging for what seemed like an eternity, I would discover money in the hole….large piles of coins of all denominations. I would bury my hands in the coins, grab as much as I could hold, lift my arms over my head and allow the coins to cascade down over me. In my dream, I never spent any of the money. I only played with it and enjoyed having it. We like having money. It makes us happy.

Although most of us are not money crazy, we do rejoice when it's not a struggle to pay the bills. There is nothing wrong with that. But do we rejoice as much in obeying God's commands? The Psalmist in Psalm 119:14 was ecstatic with the privilege of serving God: *"I rejoice in following your statutes as one rejoices in great riches."* The Message Bible dramatically expresses Psalm 112:1 this way, *"Hallelujah! Blessed man, blessed woman, who fear God, who cherish and relish his commandments."*

We normally don't think of "rejoicing" or "being blessed" in following commands. We don't "cherish and relish" rules and regulations. We tend to think of them as burdensome - something that takes away our fun. We rejoice in doing what WE want to do. We don't "cherish and relish" someone else making decisions for us. We would rather be our own bosses. If we consider the fact that our God is so much wiser and stronger than we are and His love for us is deeper than our wildest imagination, why wouldn't we trust Him to direct our paths? His commands were written to give us MORE joy, not less. Is our greatest delight in God's commands or in a delightful treat at the Dairy Queen? Do our hearts rejoice in pleasing the Lord or in pleasing ourselves?

God's decisions for us will always result in our greater good. Therefore we can celebrate our good fortune because God is on our side. We may even feel like dancing and laughing. When we submit to His will, it will give us cause to "rejoice in great riches!"

> Celestial spirit that doth roll the heart's sepulchral stone away, be this our resurrection day, the singing Easter of the soul - O gentle Master of the Wise, teach us to say: I will arise.
> ~ Richard Le Gallienne (1866 - 1947)

**FOOD FOR THOUGHT**

~ How much do I cherish and relish God's commands?

~ In what ways, as a Christian, do I feel rich?

~ How often do I feel like rejoicing in the great riches God has given me?

## SPOILED

Do you search for ways to spoil those you love with the perfect gifts for birthdays and holidays? I have a husband who spoils me – not only with gifts, but with dedicated service.

Early in our married life, I discovered I had to be extremely careful what I complained about because my husband is a man of action. He is always looking for ways to take care of me and if he thinks I have a need, he will do all he can to help. If it's 10:30 at night and I mention that I forgot to buy something at the store…..before I even realize what is happening…..he has his coat on, heading out the door.

When I am cooking in the kitchen, he will appear every so often and clean up behind me….rinsing dishes, emptying potato peelings out of the sink, and setting the table. Of course there are some slight disadvantages to this. If I reach for my stirring spoon, I may find it is already in the dishwasher or if I reach for the salt shaker, it may already be back in the cupboard. After the meal, he is right beside me helping clean up. Yes, my husband spoils me. Is my husband perfect? No, he has his share of faults along with other husbands, but his good points far exceed the not-so-good.

Are you spoiled? We are not all fortunate enough to have a person in our lives that looks out for our needs and desires. Some of us have learned to fend for ourselves and have learned it well! But we ALL have a God who spoils us! He is the One who invented the word "generosity". Why else would He have created all the beauty in the world around us? We love color but God could have created the world in black and white and we would be none the wiser. Since we rebelled against Him, He could have left us in our sin, but *"God so loved the world that he gave his only begotten Son, that whoever believes in him should not perish but have everlasting life."* (John 3:16) What a precious gift!

Is my husband helpful and generous because I am a perfect human being? Not by a long shot! Did God choose to be a giving God because we deserved it? Not by a long shot! It was a gift of grace. Does my husband spoil me because he can't help himself? No. He does it by choice. He chose to love me. He chose to marry me. He chose to be committed to me.

God made a choice as well. He chose to create us. He chose to love us. God chose to be committed to us. No matter how many times we fail Him…He invites us to return to Him. Our God spoils us!

If we allow that spoiling to create a love relationship, we will never be "spoiled rotten." It's okay for someone or Someone to spoil us if it results in a grateful, reciprocating heart.

> Lord, you are the faithful God who keeps covenant and steadfast love with those who love you and keep your commandments, to a thousand generations. You are here with me, a mighty One who will save. You rejoice over me with gladness and quiet me with your love. ~ based on Deuteronomy 7:9 & Zephaniah 3:17

**FOOD FOR THOUGHT**

~ If God gave me the perfect gift, what would it be?

~ Do I have a tendency to be under-appreciative when someone or Someone spoils me?

~ What kind of love relationship do I have with God?

## THE COLD DRIZZLES OF LIFE

When our son, Bruce, was a baby, I took him with me on a Christmas shopping trip at Dillard's Department Store in a large shopping center. Evidently I paid little attention that I had used the north door to enter the store. When I exited the store, I used the West door. For obvious reasons, I was confused and could not find my car in the parking lot.

Normally, it would not have been a big deal to experience a little delay in locating my car, but I did not have a stroller and my back was beginning to ache from carrying a healthy ten-month-old baby boy on my hip and heavy packages dangling from my arms as I wandered through the endless aisles of parked cars. Adding insult to injury, the skies began to unleash a cold, heavy drizzle of rain. Little Bruce was vehemently telling the world with a loud wail that he was not comfortable. It was not long before my own warm, salty tears began to mingle with the cold rain on my face as I continued to search for the lost car.

A kindly security guard discovered me in my wanderings through the parking lot. He put us in his vehicle and drove around to locate my car, surely saving me from a mental breakdown. The problem may have been drastically reduced had I planned ahead by bringing a stroller. Or perhaps had I not been so caught up in the moment and had been more directionally aware of my surroundings, it may have saved the day.

As we go through life, we can't stop the icy rain from falling from the sky. But we can certainly plan ahead, minimizing potential problems. We can plan ahead for our healthy lifestyle as well, deciding in advance what we will eat and how much. We can ensure that the right foods are available at the right time. If we know we are going to a buffet, we can mentally decide to limit our intake to healthy portions of nutritious foods.

No, we can't always prevent situations that bring on the warm, salty tears but by opening our eyes and being aware of our surroundings and especially our own limitations, we can shorten their duration. In our quest for a healthy lifestyle, we can be aware of the nutritional and caloric content of foods so we can make wise choices. We can be aware of our own "danger zones" and "trigger foods" that require extra precaution. We can be more aware of the arrows of temptation Satan shoots in our direction.

When the cold drizzles of life come (and they will!) we can remember that Jesus is our Good Shepherd and will do far more than the kindly Security Guard to rescue us from our plight. We don't always plan ahead. We don't always pay attention to where we are going. But Jesus is in the rescue business and He loves us. He said: *"I am the good shepherd; I know my sheep and my sheep know me - just as the Father knows me and I know the Father - and I lay down my life for the sheep."* (John 10:14-15)

> Good Shepherd, thank you for rescuing me. I praise you for being my Rock, my Fortress, my Deliverer, my Shield, my Stronghold, my Refuge and my Savior. ~ based on 2 Samuel 22:2-3

**FOOD FOR THOUGHT**

~ How well do I plan ahead?

~ In my planning, do I take into account my own limitations?

~ In what ways does God rescue me on a daily basis?

# GETTING THE AXE

When my husband, Jack, was in second grade, he received what he considered to be the best Christmas gift ever - his own axe. It was a beautiful axe with a cream-colored handle, painted blue on the end. Most of all, it was his very own. He couldn't wait to go outside and cut up wood for kindling from the slabs that came from the sawmill.

Another thing he loved during his grade school years were the boots that had a holder on the side for his jackknife. In the early 1940's, a jackknife was considered a status symbol. My husband would walk around proudly with his britches tucked inside the boots and his jackknife within handy reach.

I was also the proud owner of a jackknife in grade school. At outside recess, we girls played a game of splits. We stood facing our opponent and took turns throwing the jackknife into the ground. Holding the knife by the blade end, we threw it hard with a snap of the wrist creating a spin and hopefully making it stick in the ground close to where it was aimed. Wherever it stuck, that's where the opponent had to place her foot. The object was to throw it gradually wider each time so that the other person eventually had to do the splits. The first person to fall over lost the game.

Times have changed a great deal since the 1940's and 1950's. Today, we wouldn't think of gifting small children with weapons or allow them to take a knife to school. There is "zero tolerance" for that. But it was the farthest thing from our young minds to hurt someone else with our "weapon". It was simply a toy - a status symbol. We had no idea it could be a threat to our safety.

Perhaps its time to incorporate an attitude of "zero tolerance" for some of the weapons in our lives that threaten our physical and spiritual health. These weapons are those we play with but don't consider dangerous. We think of them as status symbols to showcase our abundance or exciting toys to be used for the enjoyment of life.

There is one weapon that is extremely dangerous - the weapon of overindulgence. It could be overindulgence in food, television or even spending. As with any weapon, the longer we play with it, the more chance there is for danger.

God is calling us to practice "zero tolerance." *"We know that our old self was crucified with him so that the body of sin might be done away with, that we should no longer be slaves to sin - because anyone who has died has been freed from sin."* (Romans 6:6-7) It's time for our tendency to overindulge to "get the axe!" Then God can make us whole and holy - spirit, soul and body - a great Christmas gift indeed!

> Help me not to be gullible, Lord. May I check out everything and keep only what's good. Make me whole and holy - spirit, soul and body - and keep me fit for your coming.
> ~ based on 1 Thessalonians 5:21,23 (MSG)

## FOOD FOR THOUGHT

~ What dangerous games am I playing with my health?

~ Which one would God most prefer to "get the axe"?

~ How do I become whole and holy, spirit, soul and body?

# THANK GOODNESS

On the way to church, we were stopped at a red light with a police car beside us on the left in a left turn lane. On our right, a car suddenly whizzed through the red light. My husband said: "He'd better watch out. That policeman will get him." No sooner were the words out of his mouth than the siren went on, the policeman cut in front of us and raced after the offender, catching him about a block away. How many times have we seen someone break the law and proclaimed, "Where is a policeman when you need him?" It felt good to see justice done.

Our son, Bruce, was working late one night. As he was coming home at 1 A.M., he stopped at a red light on a deserted country road and thought: "There is not another car within miles and I'm tired. I'm not going to sit here and wait. I'll just go through the light." After proceeding, he discovered that there WAS someone within miles. You guessed it - a policeman! Bruce did not enjoy paying the ticket. To this day, he has no clue where the policeman was hiding.

I got a ticket once too. In Indianapolis, I was driving my co-workers to a restaurant for lunch. I had forgotten my driving glasses and as I made a left turn, I thought I saw a sign out of the corner of my eye. I asked one of the girls if that was a "No Left Turn" sign. She looked back and replied, "No, it couldn't be. That policeman is turning too."

Our son-in-law, Jim, was stopped by a policeman for speeding. Although Jim did receive a ticket, he said the officer treated him with the utmost respect and kindness. Jim's reaction:

> Now THAT was interesting. I was never more calm – although not "happy" – about being stopped by the police. But what hit me was that, afterward on the way home, I was more interested in driving under the speed limit not out of an interest to be

lawful but, more so, to honor the kind police officer, and so I did. A very interesting turn of events it was, and a very nice, young police officer he was!

Some of us have had similar experiences. We could probably write a book and entitle it, "OOPS!" In our spiritual journey, we disobey God's laws for many reasons - carelessness, ignorance, disrespect, rebellion or even apathy. It's easier to figure out why we disobey than to analyze what gives us the desire to obey. Romans 2:4, however, gives us a clue. It says, *"Do you show contempt for the riches of his kindness, tolerance and patience, not realizing that God's kindness leads you toward repentance?"*

God's rules, regulations and punishments do not always inspire us to obey. It is His love, compassion, tolerance, patience, mercy and kindness toward all He has created that stirs our hearts to want to please Him. God is good! Psalms 145:9 tells us: *"The Lord is good to all; he has compassion on all he has made."*

"Thank goodness" for God's goodness!

> O God, you are my God, earnestly I seek you; my soul thirsts for you, my body longs for you, in a dry and weary land where there is no water. I have seen you in the sanctuary and beheld your power and your glory. Because your love is better than life, my lips will glorify you. I will praise you as long as I live, and in your name I will lift up my hands. My soul will be satisfied as with the richest of foods; with singing lips my mouth will praise you.
> ~ Psalm 63:1-5

### FOOD FOR THOUGHT

~ Am I really convinced God is good?

~ What inspires me to obey God?

~ When do I feel God's compassion the most?

## GOING THROUGH THE MOTIONS

When my husband and I lived in the Upper Peninsula of Michigan, we found the winter weather very "refreshing." His hometown of Newberry can reach temperatures of 30 below zero and the record one-day snowfall is 15 feet. As idealistic parents of two small children, we felt it was our duty to teach them to appreciate God's great outdoors so we decided to take them on a winter picnic.

Our first task was to bundle up the kids and ourselves with so many winter clothes that movement was next to impossible. My husband and I donned snowshoes and pulled the kids across the field on a toboggan into the woods. We rolled the kids off the toboggan and attempted to stand them upright. After wrapping thick scarves around our noses and mouths as a shield from the biting wind, we built a fire and dangled ham steaks on the end of a stick over the flame, all the while trying to convince ourselves and the kids how much fun we were having. We would eventually give up, eat cold ham and head for home as quickly as possible. By the time we arrived home, icicles dangled from our noses and we could feel nothing but numbness inside our boots and mittens.

We thought we were having fun. The truth of the matter was that we were only "going through the motions" of having fun. If we really wanted to enjoy ourselves, we should have made popcorn and played Candy Land by the fireplace. Instead, we allowed ourselves the thrill of becoming chilled to the bone.

When we are chilled to the bone, it doesn't seem possible we will ever be warm again. The summer memories of the sun sitting warm on our shoulders quickly fade to distant, almost inaccessible memories. Bodily chills are not pleasant, but even more unpleasant are the spiritual chills we may experience when we find ourselves going through the motions of religion instead of experiencing a real relationship with Jesus Christ. We attend church, read our Bibles and say our prayers. If we are doing these things out of duty rather than from a joyous response to our loving Creator, our spiritual life rapidly grows cold. We may try to simulate a past memory of the spiritual warmth that was once ours but the more we choose to follow our own desires instead of God's, the more we find ourselves chilled to the spiritual bone.

Whether we are attempting to entertain children or deepen our spiritual life, we must make an honest evaluation on whether our efforts are producing the desired results or whether we are simply fooling ourselves. The Pharisees in the Bible were only going through the motions of religion. They replaced God's tradition with the tradition of men. Jesus told His listeners, "...*But do not do what they do, for they do not practice what they preach.*" (Matthew 23:3)

To have a warm, vibrant relationship with the living God, we need to face the truth instead of just "going through the motions."

> Heavenly Father, help me to make every effort to add to my faith goodness; and to goodness, knowledge; and to knowledge, self-control; and to self-control, perseverance; and to perseverance, godliness; and to godliness, brotherly kindness; and to brotherly kindness, love.   ~ based on 2 Peter 1:5-8

**FOOD FOR THOUGHT**

~ Do I practice what I preach?

~ Could I use the words "warm and vibrant" to describe my relationship with God?

~ In which part of my spiritual journey am I tempted to "go through the motions"?

## COMMON SENSE

It was the Christmas holidays, 1958. I was attending Olivet Nazarene University in Bourbonnais, Illinois and I was the only one in my dorm not scheduled to go home for Christmas. I braced myself for the experience of ten lonely, boring days. That day I was thrilled to receive money in the mail from my mother for bus fare to her new home in Newberry, Michigan. When I arrived up north, not realizing the temperature difference and wanting to look stylish, I stepped off the bus into a deep snow bank wearing high heels.

It was Christmas morning, 1966. We had written a letter to Santa requesting that he come early because Christmas Day seemed our best option for leaving our home to begin our new life in Columbus, Ohio. Santa was pleased to oblige and our children enjoyed getting their presents early. We left Christmas morning, pulling a large U-Haul trailer with all our belongings. Later that day we stopped for lunch. As we walked into the restaurant at a Holiday Inn, every eye seemed to be upon us. We were confused by all the attention but it soon dawned on us that, although this was just an ordinary travel day for us, it was actually Christmas Day. Everyone in the restaurant was dressed in their finest attire and we, in stark contrast, were dressed in jeans and sweatshirts.

It was Christmas Day, 1970. Our 8-year-old daughter, Rhonda, was delighted to find an Easy Bake Oven under the tree! She couldn't wait to use it. Our 11-year-old son, Bruce, was equally delighted to receive a set of dumbbells! Anxious to show off his muscles, he immediately lifted them high over his head, falling backyards on top of Rhonda's pink Easy Bake Oven, breaking off the handle. It still worked well enough to make scrumptious little cakes and muffins, but it just wasn't the same.

Common sense says that stepping off a bus into a snow bank wearing high heels is not wise. Common sense says that sweatshirts and prime rib do not belong together on Christmas Day. Common sense says strength should be built up gradually before attempting to lift the maximum amount of weights in a weight set.

Common sense is sometimes not all that common. Another word for common sense in the Bible is Wisdom. Proverbs 4:6-7 tells us, *"Do not forsake wisdom, and she will protect you; love her, and she will watch over you. Wisdom is supreme; therefore get wisdom. Though it cost all you have, get understanding."*

We need wisdom to control our eating. Common sense says gaining excess weight can put more strain on the knees and heart, and increases the risk of diabetes. I have heard that every additional pound of body weight puts three extra pounds of force on the knees, every 2.2 pounds gained gives a 1% increased risk of a heart attack, and a weight gain of 10-15 pounds doubles the risk of developing type 2 diabetes.

May your life be filled with the blessings and rewards of common sense and wisdom!

---

Grant me, O Lord my God, a mind to know you, a heart to seek you, wisdom to find you, conduct pleasing to you, faithful perseverance in waiting for you and a hope of finally embracing you.   ~ St. Thomas Aquinas (1225 - 1274)

---

**FOOD FOR THOUGHT**

~ How common is common sense?

~ Do I consider myself to be a person who uses common sense?

~ How does wisdom protect me and watch over me?

## SWEAT EQUITY

Our granddaughter, Jackie, has loved to read since she was a little tyke. No matter the time of day, if she had a choice, she would have her nose in a book. I used to be concerned that when I would hand her something to read, she would skim it quickly and put it down. I handed her one of the poems I had written one time and it seemed to me that she barely glanced at it. I grinned at her and said, "Jackie, whether you like my poetry or not, you should at least pretend to read it to please me." She said, "Grandma, I *did* read it. It's good."

Then I went to an Evelyn Wood Reading Dynamics Seminar which teaches speed reading and comprehension. The average person reads anywhere from 200 to 400 words per minute. The course advertises that it is possible to double that speed. They say people can learn to read as fast as they can think. (Maybe that's my problem. I just don't think fast enough.) I spent two days working hard in the class and although my reading speed was not doubled, I was pleased as punch with my progress.

When I got home, I decided to show off a little bit to my granddaughter. Although she had not taken the course, I gave her the timed reading test complete with comprehension questions at the end. She managed to effortlessly make my score look like that of a kindergarten student. Then it dawned on me that all those times she had picked up a paper full of words and put it back down, she was actually absorbing all the material.

We all have different talents. Some of us have to work much harder than others to get the same results in some areas. Does it seem to you that dieting is a whole lot easier for some people than for others? Some people simply make a decision to lose that five pounds they gained over the holidays and before you know it, it's gone. We all find it tempting to have a pity party when others seem to manage their weight with minimal effort and it seems that we have to invest two pounds of sweat and tears for every pound we lose.

It's helpful to remember that Jesus was tempted just as we are. Satan tempted him three times and all three times He used God's Word to stop Satan in his tracks. It may seem to us that Jesus had an easy time resisting temptation because He was God. I don't think so. I think each temptation was real. Even before the temptation came, Jesus fixed in His mind the issue of obedience to His Father. In John 14:31 Jesus said: *"...the world must learn that I love the Father and that I do exactly what my Father has commanded me."* Can we say the same?

I will always struggle with my weight. It will always require the investment of "sweat equity" on my part to take the pounds off and keep them off. I will probably never get to the point where keeping my earthly temple healthy and fit comes easily, but I am finding that aiming for joyful obedience to the Lord makes life an exciting, rewarding adventure as opposed to the misery of trying to balance on the fence between pleasing self and pleasing God.

> Not to us, O LORD, not to us but to your name be the glory, because of your love and faithfulness. ~ Psalm 115:1

**FOOD FOR THOUGHT**

~ How much "sweat equity" am I willing to invest to please God?

~ What things seem harder for me to accomplish than for others?

~ What is the best way to convert my dutiful obedience to joyful obedience?

# I HATE SNAKES

I remember the time our son, David, age 12, brought home some baby snakes in a pail. He proudly showed them to us. My husband quickly informed him that they were copperheads and baby venomous snakes are quite capable of causing death.

Another time our children were swimming in the middle of the river behind our house. Although the river was not deep, our youngest daughter, Kerry, was not yet a good swimmer and too short to stand upright in the river comfortably. One of the older children carried her to the middle of the river to a large sand bar where she could enjoy the water safely. I was watching from my kitchen window when suddenly they all began screaming and exiting the river – all, that is, except Kerry, who was left wailing hysterically in the middle of the river. Evidently they saw a water snake swimming nearby. I rushed outside and coerced one of the children to rescue their sister immediately, snake or no snake!

Satan is depicted as a snake in Genesis. Snakes are deceptive. They camouflage themselves and blend in with their environment. Satan is deceptive as well. The Bible tells us he often masquerades as an angel of light. Snakes are persistent and patient. They will lie quietly for hours waiting for their prey. We cannot yell "Boo" and expect a snake to leave town. They may slither away but they'll be back. Satan is the same way. He may leave but he will be back. When Satan tempted Jesus in the wilderness, Jesus quoted scripture to defeat him. But the Bible tells us that "*When the devil had finished all this tempting, he left him until an opportune time.*" (Luke 4:13) In other words, he wasn't giving up.

Snakes can be vicious. There is a poisonous viper in Africa called the Gaboon. These snakes have two-inch long fangs and can grow to well over six feet. Its bite can kill a full grown human within 15 minutes. Satan can also be vicious. If we look at the casualties in our world, we know that Satan does not possess a gentle side. We have an abundance of individuals trapped in things such as substance abuse, dishonesty, corruption and sexual immorality. We are even finding an increase of sins against the body, which include anorexia, bulimia and obesity.

The Bible says, *"Be self-controlled and alert. Your enemy the devil prowls around like a roaring lion looking for someone to devour."* (I Peter 5:8). But there's good news! Jesus defeated Satan on the cross! "*...By embracing death, taking it into himself, he destroyed the Devil's hold on death.*" (Hebrews 2:14- MSG)

Yes, "I hate snakes." That includes Satan. When we encounter temptations, it is sometimes best to run as fast as we can in the opposite direction. Other times God expects us to fearlessly march into the river of life, snake or no snake, and claim what is rightfully ours.

> You have commanded me, Lord, to be strong and courageous. I will not be discouraged because you are with me wherever I go. You did not give me a spirit of timidity, but a spirit of power, of love and of self-discipline.
> ~ based on Joshua 1:9 and 2 Timothy 1:7

**FOOD FOR THOUGHT**

~ When I look at my community, where do I see the results of Satan's deception?

~ Am I more courageous or less courageous than I used to be?

~ Am I ready to march into the river, snake or no snake, and claim what is mine?

## TOO BLIND TO SEE

We took our family to a piano concert one time performed by Ken Medema, a well-known blind pianist who performs worldwide. He began playing the piano when he was five years old and three years later began taking lessons in classical music through Braille music instruction. He eventually began performing and recording his own songs and has published a total of 26 albums.

Our son, Bruce, age nine, was sitting up front. Ken Medema turned toward the audience and asked, "How many of you have had piano lessons? If so, let me see your hands!" Our son's hand shot in the air so quickly it looked as though it were spring loaded. As soon as he realized that his was the only hand in the air and remembered that Ken Medema could see nothing, he sheepishly lowered it, hoping no one would notice. Ken could tell by the audience's reaction that someone had raised their hand, so he enjoyed milking the episode to entertain the audience at Bruce's expense.

I recently read Fanny Crosby's biography by Bernard Ruffin. Born in 1820, Fanny was blind from the age of six weeks old. She was probably the most prolific hymnist in history, writing over 8,000 hymns. She never viewed her blindness as a handicap because she had complete trust in her Savior. The lyrics below were written in 1875.

> All the way my Savior leads me;
> What have I to ask beside?
> Can I doubt His tender mercy,
> Who through life has been my Guide?
> Heav'nly peace, divinest comfort,
> Here by faith in Him to dwell!
> For I know, whate'er befall me,
> Jesus doeth all things well;
> For I know, whate'er befall me,
> Jesus doeth all things well.

Fanny Crosby fully believed that cheerfulness was a choice. In her hymn Blessed Assurance, written in 1873, she writes:

> Perfect submission, all is at rest
> I in my Savior am happy and blessed,
> Watching and waiting, looking above,
> Filled with His goodness, lost in His love.

Fanny Crosby could "see" better than most of us!

In 2 Kings, Chapter 6, Elisha's servant was terrified to see an army with chariots surrounding the city. Elisha prayed for his servant, *"O Lord, open his eyes so he may see."* God opened the servant's eyes, and he looked and saw the hills full of horses and chariots of fire all around Elisha. Help was there all along, but the servant had limited spiritual eyesight.

Blindness comes in many forms. What we consider blindness may sometimes simply be a stubborn refusal to open our eyes to the truth. We prefer to be blind because if we don't see the problem, perhaps we can ignore our responsibility to fix it.

Are we "too blind to see"? My prayer today is that God will open our eyes to our responsibility to take good care of the marvelous bodies God gave us.

> Praise be to you, O LORD; teach me your decrees. Open my eyes that I may see wonderful things in your law. ~ Psalm 119:12,18

### FOOD FOR THOUGHT

~ How limited is my spiritual eyesight?

~ To what truth do I tend to close my eyes and ignore?

~ Do I choose to be cheerful?

# TASTE AND SEE

When we lived in Lusby, Maryland, I took care of two boys, Freddy, age 8, and Andy, age 6. Since their mother was a nurse, they were sometimes at our house on Sundays. One Sunday evening we took them to church for a special program that included a church potluck dinner. Since my husband and I had charge of the program and needed to talk briefly with our guest speaker, we sent the boys through the potluck serving line by themselves. They had never been to a potluck before so I gave them explicit instructions. I told them it was a simple procedure – just decide which foods were appealing and use the serving spoon to put a little of each on their plates.

My husband and I were standing at the back of the room talking with our guest when I happened to look up and observe the boys going through the food line. To my horror, I saw Andy use the serving spoon to put a small portion of food on his plate (just as I had instructed him) but proceeded to put the spoon in his mouth and lick it off before returning it to the bowl. Although it seemed as though I moved with the speed of lightning, he managed to lick off three serving spoons and return them to their respective bowls before I could reach him.

It was definitely improper etiquette but one thing was for sure – Andy knew what everything tasted like. He knew what was good and what, perhaps, was not. He didn't need to ask for anyone else's opinion. He had tasted it for himself.

There is a Bible verse that tells us to taste. Psalm 34:8 says, *"Taste and see that the Lord is good; blessed is the man who takes refuge in him."* We hear many testimonies on the goodness of God. We hear multiple sermons proclaiming His goodness. But until we taste for ourselves, we will never know. It's hard to explain to someone what ice-cream tastes like if he or she has never had it. We can describe it as cold, sweet, creamy or any number of adjectives, but until we convince them to take a spoonful and put it into their mouths, they will not have a clue.

Have you tasted the goodness of God? It comes in many flavors. Baskin-Robbins is well-known for its "31 flavors" slogan. They want you to "Count the Flavors. Where flavor counts." Anyone can sample a flavor with a small pink spoon. The flavors of God's goodness are so numerous, they are impossible to count. There is the goodness of His faithfulness, His grace, His mercy and His love, just to name a few. The wonderful part is that God doesn't give us a sample in a little pink plastic spoon. He doesn't tantalize us with nibble-sized blessings of His goodness. He has sufficient and He longs to share generously with us. It is never too little.

If we allow God to bless us with His goodness, body, soul and spirit, we will be able to say, "It is enough!" God satisfies! All we need to do is "taste and see."

> When your words came, I ate them; they were my joy and my heart's delight, for I bear your name, O LORD God Almighty.
> ~ Jeremiah 15:16

## FOOD FOR THOUGHT

~ Am I taking someone's word for God's goodness or have I experience it myself?

~ What does victory taste like?

~ Is the flavor of God's love satisfying to me or do I crave other things?

## COMPLETING THE CIRCUIT

In the 1980's I worked for Leaseway Transportation as the first shift supervisor of the Data Processing Center. One Thursday night I received a call at midnight from the Comptroller of the company. Evidently the third shift employees all called in sick and the Comptroller decided he would go in and print the payroll checks to meet the Friday deadline. The only problem was that he had never done it before and could not get the printer to work. I did not relish the thought of getting dressed and going in to work and, since it was a relatively simple procedure, I decided I could talk him through it over the phone.

I spent the next 45 minutes telling him how to access the computer files, which buttons to push and how to line up the checks in the printer. He still could not get the checks to print. It finally dawned on me that I had not told him to press the "on" button, assuming he had already done so. What a difference it makes when we connect to the power source to complete the circuit!

Many of the struggles and challenges we experience in life, including our disposition toward self-indulgence, stem from our ignorance on how to properly complete our spiritual circuit. We come to church or Bible Study and learn a few new things that give us fresh confidence in our Christian walk – and that's a good thing. But then we charge forward thinking we now have the proper knowledge and the right formulas that will guarantee our spiritual growth. We neglect to stay connected to the Source. Have you ever tried to explain something to someone only to be quickly interrupted with, "Yes, I know!" That's what we do to God. He has so much more to say, but we cut Him off before we have fully received all He wants to give us.

The "on" button was not hidden nor out of the Comptroller's reach. It was nearby, completely accessible. He could have used one finger and pressed it at any time. It was simply not a part of his perceived solution and was overlooked. God, also, is not hidden from us nor is He out of our reach. He is only a prayer away and He makes sure His Word is accessible to us as well. *"Now what I am commanding you today is not too difficult for you or beyond your reach. No, the word is very near you; it is in your mouth and in your heart so you may obey it."* (Deuteronomy 30:11, 14)

Through God's Word and through prayer, we can reach out and touch Him at any time. The incomprehensible part is when we overlook Him as the Ultimate Solution. Whatever we lack, He can provide. Whether we lack persistence, courage, faith, self-control, self-confidence, wisdom or even companionship, He is the Ultimate Provider.

Pressing our spiritual "on" button means saying "yes" to the Father. Completing our spiritual circuit means spending a lifetime learning how to become "one" with the Father and with His purposes.

---

Jehovah Jireh, you supply all my needs according to your riches in glory. Help me to stay connected to you because every good and perfect gift comes from above.
~ based on Philippians 4:19 & James 1:17

---

**FOOD FOR THOUGHT**

~ Am I connected to the Source?

~ Which of my self-absorbed tendencies have created breaks in the spiritual line?

~ Which spiritual characteristic do I seem to lack?

# SERVICE WITH A SMILE

The first Wednesday of every month is Senior Citizens' Day at Kroger's. Since they offer seniors a 10% discount, the grocery aisles are always filled to the max with elderly shoppers. In addition to saving money, seniors now have an added blessing. A group of volunteers faithfully appear at Kroger's each month on the first Wednesday to assist seniors where needed. They sanitize grocery carts, help locate hard-to-find items, unload groceries onto the checkout counter and load purchased groceries into the car.

The volunteers wear bright lime-green t-shirts with the name "A.C.T.S." (Acknowledging Christ Through Service.) "A.C.T.S." is the brainstorm of Tracy Harlan, Children's Pastor of 1$^{st}$ Church of God in Marion. She explained to me that God inspired her through an evangelist at camp who emphasized the need to go outside the walls of the church to "show them Jesus."

Each month, 10 or 15 members of 1$^{st}$ Church of God set aside the many responsibilities and obligations of their own lives for the purpose of sharing their time and energy with others to "show them Jesus." And...they do it with a smile! The smile comes easily because they are not serving out of obligation, but from the heart. It is a smile that reflects the love of Jesus for every person God created.

We, too, are called to "show them Jesus!" We are all called to "Acknowledge Christ Through Service." Jesus tells us in Matthew 25:40: *"...I tell you the truth, whatever you did for one of the least of these brothers of mine, you did for me."* And...we are called to do it with a smile! I'm wondering about the true value of a service that cannot be done with a smile. It reduces the task to an obligation, a chore, a duty or a burden.

I joined a small group sponsored by our church called "The Mayberry Bible Study." It helped us search for gospel truths in the

Andy Griffith television series. Where can a television show be found today that is so family friendly and includes a moral lesson in every episode? Lesson One zeroed in on the "heavenly purpose of earthly service." We observed many practical examples of a small town sheriff who consistently put the needs of his community above his own. Andy Griffith gave "service with a smile."

The Bible is clear: *"If anyone has material possessions and sees his brother in need but has no pity on him, how can the love of God be in him? Dear children, let us not love with words or tongue but with actions and in truth."* (I John 3:17, 18) Yes, we are called to serve others, but we can serve others better if we take care of ourselves. If we care for our physical bodies by choosing the proper proportions of food, exercise and rest, we will have the health and energy necessary to serve those in need.

"Service with a smile" is our joyful privilege whether we are serving God by assisting others or serving God by caring for the wonderful bodies He designed and created.

> Lord, Open my eyes to the needs of others for this is the service you have chosen - to loose the chains of injustice, set the oppressed free, share my food with the hungry, provide for the poor, and clothe the naked. Then my light will break forth like the dawn and your glory will be my rear guard. ~ based on Isaiah 58:6-8

## FOOD FOR THOUGHT

~ Do I give service with a smile?

~ What is the heavenly purpose of earthly service?

~ How did I show love with action this past week?

## THE DEFUSER

When my husband, Jack, encounters a grouchy salesperson, he takes it on as a personal challenge to get him or her to smile before we leave the store. Since he can be quite witty, he is usually successful. There is one clerk in a small store who always seemed to be moody. We now find him chatting amiably with us every time we come. I'd like to think that a large amount of the credit is due to my husband's efforts.

The world in which we live has an overabundance of grouchy people. I'd rather not include myself in that statistic because I can usually see the bright side of things. One day, however, I found myself growing grouchier by the minute in the saga of buying a new upright vacuum cleaner. We found one we liked but it came with expensive cloth filter bags. We told the salesman we wanted to buy this particular vacuum cleaner only if paper replacement bags were available. He assured us they were and sold us a set of paper bags with the vacuum. But a couple weeks later when we tried to change the bag, we discovered they were designed for a canister vacuum cleaner.

No problem. We would just go back to the store (trip #2) and exchange them. When we arrived, we were told by a different salesman that the cloth replacement bags were the only ones available for that vacuum cleaner. We were not convinced so we returned home and called the factory. The factory gave us the code number for the replacement bags. So we went back to the store (trip #3) only to find out that the factory had given us the code number for the cloth bag. A 3rd salesman reaffirmed there were no paper bags available.

We went home and put the vacuum cleaner in the trunk intending to return it. We marched back to the store (trip # 4), ready to talk with a manager and demand the right to return the vacuum. But salesman #4 promised he could be of help. He was so gentle, so compassionate, so kind and so reassuring that all my anxiety was quickly defused. He gave us the proper bags (with a smile) at no extra charge. My irritation drained away like dirty water down a bathtub drain.

There are many things in this life that hit us between the eyes. How many times do we allow our circumstances to affect our attitude? Our mood swings affect us in negative ways, which can include yielding to the temptation to reach for comfort foods when we are not hungry.

How much greater is God's ability to defuse our anxiety when and if we come to him! He is so gentle, so compassionate, so kind and so reassuring that all our anxiety quickly melts in the warmth of His love. 1 Peter 5:7 tells us exactly how and why it works... *"Cast all your anxiety on him because he cares for you."* We have no excuse to be grouchy because God is The Great Defuser of everything contrary to His Kingdom.

> O Lord God Almighty, redeem my soul from its bondage that I may be free to live henceforth, not for myself, but for you. Help me to put away self, and to remember that this life is not given for my ease, my enjoyment. It is a schooling time for the eternal home you have prepared for those who love you.
> ~ Maria Hare (1798 – 1870)

## FOOD FOR THOUGHT

~ What gives me the most anxiety?

~ What works best to defuse my anger?

~ In what ways can I overcome evil with good?

## ABUNDANT LIFE

Whenever my husband received a job transfer that included a relocation to another state, he would go on ahead to purchase the new house while I stayed behind to sell the old one. He always did an excellent job of choosing houses that pleased me. We normally liked many of the same things in houses except for one. My husband is extremely conservative by nature and I delight in color and contrast. The house in Oklahoma he picked out had beige carpeting throughout and matching draperies of dusty green in every room. It was actually very becoming, but the longer we were there, the more I began to crave a splash of color.

When it came time for retirement, after much internet research, we chose Marion, Illinois as our new place of residence. Since my husband purchased all the other houses, he said it was my turn. I was thrilled. He stayed behind with my mother while I drove from Oklahoma to Southern Illinois by myself. I found a lovely three-bedroom villa that would meet our needs. I immediately fell in love with the bright yellow kitchen and saw numerous decorating possibilities for the rest of the house. After we moved in, my first project was to purchase an area rug for the laminate floors in the living room. It didn't take long at Home Depot to find exactly what I wanted – a red rug with designs that included leopards and monkeys. I added bright red swag curtains for just the right touch. I am thoroughly enjoying the splashes of color in our home and I love having monkeys in my living room.

Do you have any monkeys in your living room? Chances are, you prefer the beige carpeting and that's okay, but if we are honest with ourselves, there are areas of our lives that are more humdrum than we would like them to be. Many of us have settled into a beige, dusty green mediocre existence. As we wake up each morning and go through the same motions as the day before, we begin to long for a splash of color in our lives. Something more than mediocre. Something exciting. Something vibrant.

One of my favorite passages of scripture is found in Ezekiel, Chapter 47. I love the visual image of a great river flowing from the throne of God. The Bible tells us that when the river enters stagnant waters, the sea becomes fresh. Verse 9 says, *"where the river flows everything will live."*

I believe the river represents the flow of the Holy Spirit in us. John 7:38 (NKJV) says: *"He who believes in Me, as the Scripture has said, out of his heart will flow rivers of living water."* There is NOTHING mediocre about living water! If we find our efforts toward a healthy life-style bogged down in the humdrum, the living water will refresh our goals and aspirations.

For our satisfaction, it's not mandatory to have monkeys in our living rooms, but it is essential to allow the Spirit to flow through us, ridding us of stagnant water and filling us with "abundant life." *"Where the river flows, everything will live!"*

> Heavenly Father, sovereign Lord,
> By Your glorious Name adored!
> Faint we were, and parched with drought,
> Water at Your word gushed out,
> Streams of grace our thirst repress,
> Starting from the wilderness;
> Still we gasp Your grace to know,
> Here forever let it flow,
> Make the thirsty land a pool;
> Fix the Spirit in our soul.
> ~ Charles Wesley (1707 - 1788)

**FOOD FOR THOUGHT**

~ How vibrant and alive is my relationship with God?

~ What blocks the flow of the living water?

~ In what ways might I share the living water with others?

# LIFE PACKS A PUNCH!

I was reading a while back about Mantis Shrimp. Although they are only a few inches long, they can throw the fastest and strongest punch of any animal. They strike with the force of a rifle bullet and can even shatter aquarium glass. Mantis Shrimp use an ingenious energy storage system. When the arm is cocked, a ratchet holds it in place, then the muscles contract and build up energy. When the latch is released, all the energy is released at once, acting like a spring and accelerating up to 10,000 times the force of gravity. It really "packs a punch."

Life can be like that sometimes. Everything seems to be going well. Life is predictable, satisfactory and rewarding. Then, when we least expect it, "life packs a punch," turning our world upside down spiraling us out of control.

That's the way I felt on March 1, 2010, when my world came to an abrupt halt in an automobile accident. My husband and I were on our way to a home-based Bible Study group when our view was blocked and we unknowingly turned in front of an oncoming pick-up truck. Both my husband and I lost consciousness and sustained major injuries. Paramedics were at the scene quickly, called by good Samaritan witnesses. The fire department was called to extricate us from our car.

My husband was taken to Heartland Regional Medical Center in Marion, IL, and I was airlifted to Deaconess Hospital in Evansville, IN, which is a Level 1 Trauma Center. My husband was treated and released the next day. He had a large gash on the head and damaged back muscles. After nine days in the trauma unit, I was transferred to Shawnee Christian Nursing Center in Herrin, IL for rehabilitation. In addition to 19 stitches in the forehead, I had a broken collarbone, multiple broken ribs, a lacerated liver, a punctured lung and colorful bruises from head to toe. My recuperation has been a lengthy one, but I am blessed with almost full recovery.

What do we do when "life packs a punch?" There are obvious choices. We can give up on our goals and look to this world's coping measures of self-pity and self-indulgence, or we can open our eyes to the fact that God is in control and He will fulfill His purposes in spite of all evidence that points to the contrary.

Romans 8:28 tells us, *"We know that in all things God works for the good of those who love him, who have been called according to his purpose."* If there is one thing I have learned from this experience, it is that God is not done with me yet. In His great mercy, an accident that should have taken my life or at the very least, left me incapacitated, has instead given me a new lease on life, a renewed appreciation for the wonderful bodies He created for us, and a new sense of the privilege that is ours for serving the awesome God of the universe. That really "packs a punch!"

> O Father, when our best was not good enough, and when our highest could not reach the Kingdom, You came to lift us to yourself. What mercy. What humility. What grace. We are speechless before the wonder of it. Read our thankful hearts.
> ~ E. Stanley Jones (1884–1973)

**FOOD FOR THOUGHT**

~ Are my eyes on my circumstances or on the power of the Almighty God of the Universe?

~ What coping measures do I use when life packs a punch?

~ What can I do to show appreciation for the wonderful body God gave me?

# FRUSTRATED

Have you ever been frustrated? Chances are the answer is yes. Being frustrated can mean many things – disappointed, thwarted, dissatisfied, unresolved. Allowing ourselves to be frustrated can zap our energy and easily sidetrack us from our goals.

Frustrations in life frequently express themselves in dreams. Many years ago, as a new college student, I had a recurring dream that I was trying to get to my first day of class on time. I remember taking elevators that went nowhere. One elevator even took me up several stories and opened onto the roof. Once I found myself in a long hallway of rooms where every room had the same room number, but it was not the number I was looking for. I continually looked at my watch thinking, "Time is running out. I have to get to class before it starts."

My husband had a dream one night that he was in a play and forgot his lines. He faked it through the first act and then refused to go on stage for the second. He was happy to wake up and discover it was all a dream. Being frustrated can leave us with a sense of urgency such as my dream about getting to class on time. Or, as in my husband's dream, when our frustrations are caused by our own mistakes, we simply give up.

Many of us are frustrated in our attempts to lose weight. We gear up to get started and get an invitation to a birthday party. We eat the right things for two weeks and the scale doesn't move. We watch others eating everything we love and they don't gain a pound. It's like taking an elevator to nowhere. How many times have we been so frustrated that we wish it were a dream and we could wake up and find it gone? Of course, "wishing" doesn't solve the problem.

In the book of Ezra, God's people had returned from captivity in Babylon and were attempting to rebuild the temple. But "*the peoples around them set out to discourage the people of Judah and make them afraid to go on building. They hired counselors to work against them and frustrate their plans..."* Ezra 4:4,5  Satan knows that allowing a little frustration to creep in works best of all. Mental frustrations can be worse than physical ones.

God never leaves us hopeless and helpless!  His answer to our frustrations is found in Psalm 47:4-6.  *"Delight yourself in the Lord and he will give you the desires of your heart. Commit your way to the Lord; trust in him and he will... make our righteousness shine like the dawn, the justice of your cause like the noonday sun."*  Step number one is to "delight ourselves in the Lord." Steps two and three are to "commit our way to the Lord" and "trust in Him." God has the power to convert our worst frustrations into our best victories!

---

Father, let me not grow weary of doing good, for in due season I will reap if I do not give up. Help me to throw off everything that hinders and the sin that so easily entangles and run with perseverance the race marked out for me.
~ based on Galatians 6:9 & Hebrews 12:1

---

**FOOD FOR THOUGHT**

~ Why are mental frustrations worse than physical ones?

~ What frustrates me the most?

~ How do I delight myself in the Lord?

# WELCOME!

In the winter of 1977, my husband, Jack, moved to an apartment in Chicago to start his new job and I stayed behind in Lusby, Maryland to sell our home. When it came time for the house closing, I obtained power of attorney for my husband's signature because he was on a business trip to the United Arab Emirates. After the moving van was loaded, my two daughters, Rhonda and Kerry, and our white Cockapoo, Ginger, started the 850-mile trip to our new home.

We made plans to stay at a motel one night on the way. I had dutifully called ahead to find out if they allowed dogs. They told me, "No problem!" But when we arrived, I discovered that they had placed us on the third floor. I reminded them that we had requested the first floor because of the dog. The hotel clerk immediately shushed me and said with a look of horror, "Because of the what?!" Evidently dogs were not allowed after all and we had been misinformed.

The clerk relented and allowed us to stay the night, giving us a first-floor room, but admonished us to "keep the dog out of sight!" Hmmm. Interesting. How do you take a dog that needs to go outside down a long hallway on a leash, past a multitude of occupied rooms and keep her out of sight? So we devised a plan. I would go outside and one of my daughters would hand Ginger out the motel window and then I would hand her back in when she was done. Although I had to step over large snow banks, the plan worked perfectly.

We had to sneak our dog in and out of the building because Ginger was not a welcome guest. We feel the same way, sometimes, when we go to God in prayer. We do not feel welcome because we assume God's great displeasure with our imperfections. Nothing could be farther from the truth. God delights in His children and He loves to have us spend time with Him.

Hebrews 4:16 tells us that we are to *"...come boldly to the throne of grace, that we may obtain mercy and find grace to help in time of need."* When we are the least worthy, God throws out His extravagant "WELCOME" mat. He bids us come and share in His holiness when we have none of our own.

When we have messed up for the umpteenth time…when we have made selfish, childish choices…when we have used up our last excuse – our God, who is full of grace and mercy, throws His arms around us and breathes a fresh breath of hope into us. Ephesians 2:4 tells us why. *"Because of his great love for us, God, who is rich in mercy, made us alive with Christ even when we were dead in transgressions - it is by grace you have been saved."*

We don't need to sneak in or out of a window or go in the back door to find God. We are encouraged to come boldly to His throne. We are always "welcome" in the presence of God.

> Have mercy on me, O God, according to your unfailing love; according to your great compassion blot out my transgressions. Wash away all my iniquity and cleanse me from my sin.
> ~ Psalm 51:1-2

**FOOD FOR THOUGHT**

~ Do I feel welcome and loved in the presence of God?

~ How do I rid myself of guilt feelings for things that have already been forgiven?

~ What does it mean to come "boldly" to the throne of grace?

# FINISH THE RACE

My friend, Danielle Barter, is a jogger. She recently had an interesting experience during her jog and shares the following story:

>Today, I jogged with a goat. It saw me, ran straight for me (I thought it was going to head-butt me), then fell in beside me for a full mile, panting and bleating loudly. (Perhaps it sensed I could communicate with it since I had kissed another goat at the high school a few months ago for the FFA fundraiser.) We created quite a spectacle for the fleet of workers leaving their boss's farm. Every man among them was laughing - hard. Even funnier is the fact that one after one, the drivers of the fleet of vehicles who passed me would roll down their windows, and between belly-laughs, say, "You're jogging with a goat!" As if I hadn't already noticed!
>
>I felt bad leaving the goat behind when it could no longer keep up. That goat really needed some exercise. It was quite chunky. If it hadn't invested so much of its energy in bleating the whole time we ran, it might have been able to complete the full four miles with me, instead of giving up after one.

Danielle's "goat story" gives us cause to wonder. Where do WE expend our energy? If we choose a new diet program, do we use all our energy bleating and complaining about how difficult it is? Do we use every ounce of our strength on pity parties thinking how unfair it is that others seem to be able to achieve fitness without the sacrifices we seem to make? For some of us, our "get-up-and-go" seems to have "got-up-and-went." Maybe the reason for this is because we have allowed our energy to be used up on nonessential things.

When I lived in Maryland, several in our church came together and started a Diet Club. We met weekly and usually spent each session complaining about the difficulty we had staying on the program and crying on each other's shoulder about all the temptations we had during the week. We finally disbanded without one success story among us.

The Israelites in the Bible, (like Danielle's goat) put a great deal of energy into complaining. *"The rabble with them began to crave other food, and again the Israelites started wailing and said, 'If only we had meat to eat! We remember the fish we ate in Egypt at no cost - also the cucumbers, melons, leeks, onions and garlic. But now we have lost our appetite; we never see anything but this manna!'"* (Numbers 11:4-6) The Lord had been good to them when they had nothing to eat, providing free food in the form of manna. Yet they channeled their energy into negativity. Perhaps that's why they wandered in the desert for 40 years instead of reaching the Promise Land.

If we choose to invest our energy into bleating and complaining (like Danielle's goat), we will never complete the race God has set before us. Victory can be ours when we quit complaining and use our strength to "finish the race!"

> Lord, may I be able to say, along with the Apostle Paul... "I have fought the good fight, I have finished the race, I have kept the faith."    ~ based on 2 Timothy 4:7

**FOOD FOR THOUGHT**

~ Do I usually finish what I start?

~ What percentage of my energy is wasted in complaints?

~ Is my focus on the hardships or the finish line?

# HUNGRY?

My daughter, Rhonda, shares the following cooking experience:

MONDAY: Made a huge pot of homemade Ham and Bean soup with the Thanksgiving ham bone from the freezer. The soup burned a little, so it had that distinctive "charcoal" taste. Served with spoons and crackers.

TUESDAY: Leftover Ham and Bean soup. Decided to try cornmeal dumplings in it. I got the soup bubbling, then dropped the cornmeal batter into it. The batter disintegrated and mixed into the soup. I added the rest of it and managed to keep some of it floating to make dumplings. Not wanting to stir up what was left of the batter, I left the soup alone to bubble, thicken and burn underneath the dumplings adding to that distinctive burnt flavor. The soup was now Ham and Bean Cornmeal Mush, worthy of a fork.

WEDNESDAY: Took some hamburger from the freezer for meatloaf. Mixed a generous portion of Ham and Bean Cornmeal Mush into the meat along with some eggs and breadcrumbs. Shaped it into a pretty meatloaf. The soup was now Ham and Bean Cornmeal Mush Meatloaf with a distinctive burnt flavor.

THURSDAY: Took out some nice Tilapia from the freezer. Decided not to get creative with the fish and just baked it. Took another generous portion of Ham and Bean Cornmeal Mush, added the basic ingredients of cornbread, plopped it into a pan and stuck it in the oven. The soup was now Ham and Bean Mush Cornbread and, even though, it was as dense as a brick, it was somewhat tasty with a spread of butter on it even with that distinctive burnt flavor.

FRIDAY: Threw out the remaining Ham and Bean Cornmeal Mush, the Mush Meatloaf and the Mush Cornbread brick. After all, it's pizza night!

It's admirable to be persistent. Tenacity has always been one of Rhonda's strong characteristics. But even she admitted there comes a time when we should give up and go a different direction. It's possible to be very tenacious about the wrong things, for instance, such as persistently seeking the pleasures of this world to satisfy our spiritual needs. No matter how many things we try, it will always have that "distinctive" worldly flavor.

We look to television or movies to eliminate our boredom. We look to a beauty treatment to sooth our anxiety. We look to a shopping spree to pacify our personal dissatisfactions. We look to excess food to satisfy our spiritual hunger. Enough is enough. Some of those things are good in moderation, but were never meant to satisfy our hunger for God. It never works. The time has come to throw out what is not working and latch onto what does work. Are you hungry? Jesus told us in Matthew 5:6, *"Blessed are those who hunger and thirst for righteousness, for they will be filled."*

> Lord, teach us, whatsoever state we are in, therewith to be content; let us know both how to be abased, and how to abound; every where, and in all things, let us be instructed both to be full and to be hungry, both to abound and to suffer need; and let godliness with contentment be great gain to us; for a little, with the fear of the Lord and quietness, is better than great treasure and trouble therewith. ~ Matthew Henry (1662-1714)

## FOOD FOR THOUGHT

~ Would other people describe me as tenacious?

~ What do I do when I'm bored?

~ How do I develop a hunger and thirst for righteousness?

# ASK!

How important are questions? There is something about a question that begs to be answered. Once asked, our minds automatically begin to work toward an answer. Asking questions of ourselves can help us discover who we are and why we do what we do. Have you ever participated in a group that encouraged "brainstorming?" How does brainstorming work? It starts by asking questions such as, "If there were no limitations, how would I solve this problem?" Everyone is encouraged to share ideas, no matter how seemingly outrageous. Each question leads to other questions eventually paving the way to the right answers. There is an *unlimited* supply of good questions that lead us in the right direction. Below are a few. Add your own to the list.

Am I asking the right questions? Do I have preconceived ideas on what the answers should be or do I have an open mind? Will I recognize the answers or do I realize that the answers may come in new or unconventional ways?

What is my purpose in life? Was I created simply to be a receiver and a consumer? What are my goals in life? If I reach them, will I battle pride? If I don't reach them, will I battle self-contempt? How can I minimize self-focus in either direction and visualize a victory?

Do I want to be the best me I can be? Am I doing all I can to reflect that desire? Am I addicted to mediocrity? Am I caught in the repetitive path of least resistance?

Do I toy with sin? Do I treat it as inconsequential or do I treat it aggressively as a cancer of the soul? Do I have zero tolerance? Do I unwittingly invite sin into my life? If something is a sin, am I willing to admit it and take prompt action to correct it?

If my struggle is not against flesh and blood, what kind of weapons work best? Why did Jesus use scripture to fight temptation in the wilderness? Why is God's Word called the Sword of the Spirit? If I know the enemy is coming, do I want to be caught with no armor?

What kind of example do I set for others? Are there those who are watching me and following my example? Is that a good thing?

How grateful am I for all God's blessings? If I am grateful, will I want more than my share? Is my gratefulness based on feelings of duty or a passionate heart response? How often do I thank God for all my blessings?

Who or what do I love? Do I love people more than things? Is there any person or any thing I love more than I love God? How do I love God with heart, soul, strength and mind? Which one of those areas is the hardest for me?

*"Ask and it will be given to you; seek and you will find; knock and the door will be opened to you."* (Matthew 7:7)

> Lord, what is your will that I do? I am completely open to your plan for me. I desire to live only in you and to be guided by you forever. Grant that your holy will may be carried out perfectly in me. ~ St. Jane Frances de Chantal (1572-1641)

## FOOD FOR THOUGHT

~ In what ways do I toy with sin?

~ Do I have preconceived ideas on how God should answer my prayers?

~ Am I completely open to God's will for my life?

# ONE MAN'S TRASH

The expression, "One man's trash is another man's treasure," could very well apply to garage sales. When people decide to have a garage sale, they round up all the things they feel no longer have value or usefulness for their household and put them up for sale.

There are a lot of unusual things sold at garage sales. Believe it or not, my husband and I passed one in Clarendon Hills, Illinois one time that had a coffin for sale displayed on the front sidewalk. (I didn't ask if it was used.) I sold a "cow" one time at one of my garage sales. Our church in Mustang, Oklahoma had a program with a cowboy theme. My husband and I took a black and white Gateway computer box and made an adorable black and white square cow to use as part of the decorations. We wondered what to do with our square cow afterwards and decided to put it in our garage sale. We asked the gentleman that bought it for $3.00 what in the world he planned to do with it. He said, "I'm going to put it on my neighbor's porch, ring the doorbell and run!"

It's surprising how many go to garage sales and find something they consider valuable or desirable from other people's cast-a-ways. I love going to garage sales. My husband is of the opinion that all garage sales are full of useless junk, but I find them both a source of entertainment and an opportunity to find a great bargain. We do, however, have to be careful we are not spending our hard-earned cash for something worthless. A bargain is not a bargain if we don't need it or if the quality is questionable.

Psalm 119:37 gives us some good advice, *"Turn my eyes away from worthless things..."* There are a lot of worthless things in this world. We must constantly evaluate if we are placing too much emphasis on the worthless things of life and giving little thought to the things that truly matter. If you think about it, junk food would fit into that category. It was never God's intention that we take over-processed foods totally devoid of nutritional value, foods that destroy our health, and raise them to a high level of importance. In so doing we bypass the foods that God created. These foods, such as fresh fruits, vegetables and whole grains, are full of the nutrition that creates strong, healthy bodies. Yet we sometimes choose the foods with high sugar, salt and fat. Remember – a bargain is not a bargain if we don't need it or if the quality is questionable!

When we lived in Las Vegas, my mother accidentally put her original engagement ring in our garage sale. Fortunately my daughter spotted it before the sale started and removed it. Someone could have found a real treasure. There are times "one man's trash" could be another man's (or woman's) treasure, but we must also be careful we do not bypass the treasures God created for us and settle for trash.

> Teach me, O LORD, to follow your decrees; then I will keep them to the end. Give me understanding, and I will keep your law and obey it with all my heart. Direct me in the path of your commands, for there I find delight. Turn my heart toward your statutes and not toward selfish gain. Turn my eyes away from worthless things; preserve my life according to your word. ~ Psalm 119:33-37

**FOOD FOR THOUGHT**

~ Am I settling for things that God might consider trash?

~ How am I tempted to place too much emphasis on the things in life that have little value?

~ How do my intentions for using food differ from God's original plan?

## COVER ALL YOUR BASES

On July 14, 2009, we drove to St. Louis, Missouri to pick up our two teenage grandsons, Sam and Joe and their friend, Ezra. They were flying from Oklahoma City to spend two weeks with us in Marion, Illinois. As we drove through St. Louis on the freeway, we noticed police cars with flashing lights blocking every entrance ramp. I facetiously remarked to my husband, "Wow. The President must be coming!" It immediately dawned on us that, yes indeed, the President WAS coming. President Barak Obama was scheduled to throw out the first ball at Busch Stadium for the Major League All-Star game.

After a lengthy wait at the airport, we welcomed our teenagers. They piled into our car and we left the airport heading toward home. Once again, as we were traveling down the freeway, we observed multiple police cars with flashing lights, blocking all entrance ramps. Soon after, we passed the Presidential motorcade on the opposite side of the freeway. At least a dozen police cars, as well as some police motorcycles with lights flashing and sirens blaring, surrounded the limousine. It was quite a sight. They were taking every precaution to protect our President. They were covering all their bases, anticipating every possibility.

If the police knew the direction from which the enemy planned to come, it would have simplified everything. They would only have to close one single ramp to protect the President instead of closing ramps for several miles. Enemies never publicly announce their coming. They count on the element of surprise.

Our enemy is Satan. He counts on the element of surprise as well. If we knew which direction Satan would be coming to temp us to an unhealthy lifestyle, we would need to guard only one entrance into our hearts and minds and souls. But he is noted for his deception. In fact, in Revelation 12:9, he is called, *"the deceiver of the whole world."* Therefore, we need to "cover all our bases."

In the book of Nehemiah, God's people were attempting to rebuild the walls of Jerusalem. When their enemies heard about it, they were furious and threatened to fight against them. God's people not only prayed, they also took physical action. *"We countered with prayer to our God and set a round-the-clock guard against them."* (Nehemiah 4:9) They *"stationed armed guards at the most vulnerable places of the wall and assigned people by families with their swords, lances and bows."* (Nehemiah 4:13) They were ready! They covered all their bases.

It is the same with our temptation to lead an unhealthy life-style. Which entrance is most insecure? Where have we let down our guard? We must choose our heaviest guard at the entrances where we are most vulnerable, whether it be stress, pity parties, pleasure-seeking, etc. Don't hold back on the power! Use prayer to our God first and foremost. Then use the flashing lights and sirens of the Word of God and the Name of Jesus. We must let the enemy know we mean business. Let's cover all our bases!

> Lord Jesus, there is power in your name. You have been exalted to the highest place and your name is above every other name. At the sound of your name every knee will bow and every tongue will confess that you are Lord.   ~ based on Philippians 2:9-11

**FOOD FOR THOUGHT**

~ Does the enemy know I am serious or does he consider me a pushover?

~ When and where does the enemy find me most vulnerable?

~ How can I rid myself of the attitude of complacency?

# HEART OF A SERVANT

My husband, Jack, has a servant's heart. It was probably instilled in him from a young age by the example of his father, George Edwards. George owned and operated a small grocery store in Newberry, Michigan. No one in town ever had to go hungry. They could always come to his store and get a bag of groceries whether they had money or not. Even if they came to the house after hours, George would go to the store to get them some food. He also invested himself in many other service projects such as organizing the Lion's Club Christmas party for underprivileged children.

When we lived in Oklahoma City, my husband and I helped our church sponsor meals for the homeless through Skyline Ministries. Some of the people who came were from the nearby low-income neighborhood and some were actually homeless. There was a church service first and then we put food on tables at the back of the church. Everyone went through the serving line to get a large plateful of home-cooked food…everyone, that is, except Cheryl. She was not permitted to go through the line because of her offensive odor. Cheryl had seeping sores all over her legs and ankles, wore men's tennis shoes two sizes too big and wore every layer of clothes she owned, one on top of the other. There was always a large black gob of goo hanging from her hair that looked like bear grease. Cheryl was a "bag lady" in the true sense of the word. In fact, as soon as she arrived, the director headed up and down the aisles spraying a can of Lysol.

Cheryl sat by herself in a corner of the church and one of us had to fix her a plate and hand-deliver it. My husband always volunteered. In fact, he would stay and chat for a while. At first she was belligerent, grabbing the food and asking him to leave. But little by little he won her confidence and she began to appreciate his efforts to help.

Jesus tells us we are to be servants. He told His disciples in Mark 9:35, *"If anyone wants to be first, he must be the very last, and the servant of all."* Being a servant may mean sacrificing our own desires for the good of others. Being a servant may also mean sacrificing our own desires for the good of ourselves! Mathew Henry, who wrote an exhaustive six-volume Bible Commentary in 1706, has a powerful statement that is timeless. He said, "The body is a servant to the soul." If our body is to serve our soul, we must subordinate our flesh-desires to our spirit-desires. This is truly the meaning of the word sacrifice.

Another important element of true service is that it begins with a servant's heart, serving out of love rather than duty – serving willingly, wholeheartedly and without reservation. It is our privilege and joy to serve others and it is the privilege and joy of the body to serve the soul. It brings joy to the Father when we have the "heart of a servant!"

> Most holy, and blessed, and glorious Lord God, whose we are, and whom we are bound to serve, for because you made us, and not we ourselves, therefore we are not our own, but yours, and unto you, O Lord, do we lift up our souls. Restore us to another day in safety, and prepare us for the duties and events of it: and by all supports and comforts of this life, let our bodies be fitted to serve our souls in your service, and enable us to glorify you with both, remembering that we are not our own, we are bought with a price.
> ~ Matthew Henry (1662-1714)

**FOOD FOR THOUGHT**

~ How much energy do I expend trying to be first?

~ Am I a servant? How? Where?

~ How is my body a servant to my soul?

## TAKE REFUGE

We took the grandkids to Ray Fosse Park to play. I was sitting at a picnic bench watching them when I heard someone screaming. I looked in the direction of the scream and saw a young mother and small child backing away from a playful, fluffy, 3-month-old golden retriever puppy. Both mother and child were petrified. It was sad to see they were upset, but it was almost comical to see a grown woman fearful of a cute little ball of fur. The owner of the dog came to the rescue.

When I was 15 years old, I was home alone during Christmas break from school. My father had passed away on December 22$^{nd}$. My mother and I took a short trip after the funeral to be with relatives in Indiana, then came home and my mother returned to work. One evening, I was doing homework in our 2$^{nd}$ story apartment and everything was quiet. I went to the kitchen to sharpen a pencil, passing the stairwell that led to our apartment from a first-floor entrance. My girlfriend had snuck in the door, crept up the stairs and as I walked by, reached out and grabbed my ankle. To her delight, I gave a blood-curdling scream. She thought it was hilarious, but for some reason I failed to find the humor.

Have you ever been afraid? What makes your heart jump into your throat? A strange noise when you are alone at night? Bad news from the doctor? An unexpected financial crisis? Some fears are justified and some are unfounded, but do we know the difference? For those of us who are overweight, should we not be afraid of all the statistics we hear about the dangers of obesity?

There will always be things in life that catch us off guard, but there are times when being caught off guard is inexcusable. What is the purpose of fear? When the fear is justified, its purpose is to inspire us to make wise choices and make the necessary changes to prevent tragedy. Proverbs 22:3 says, "*A prudent person sees danger and takes refuge, but the simple keep going and suffer for it."*

According to this scripture, Step #1 is seeing the danger. Today's modern information systems give us complete and accurate statistics on the dangers of obesity. Weight-related health risks are prevalent and the information is readily available.

Step #2 is taking refuge. How do we take refuge? We can take refuge in two ways. First, we can take the necessary action to remove ourselves as far from the danger as possible. In the case of obesity, that means changing to a healthy diet and exercise program. Secondly, when we are, for whatever reason, unable to remove ourselves, we can seek refuge in the One who can. Jesus does not want us to be afraid.

When we see the danger and "take refuge," the result is safety and peace. Jesus said, *"Peace I leave with you; my peace I give you. I do not give to you as the world gives. Do not let your hearts be troubled and do not be afraid."* (John 14:27)

> Let all who take refuge in you be glad; let them ever sing for joy. Spread your protection over them, that those who love your name may rejoice in you. For surely, O LORD, you bless the righteous; you surround them with your favor as with a shield.
> ~ Psalm 5:11-12

**FOOD FOR THOUGHT**

~ Am I singing for joy or cowering in fear?

~ What is the purpose of fear?

~ How well educated am I on the dangers of an unhealthy lifestyle?

## WHAT DID YOU SAY?

In 1988, one of my co-workers at Leaseway Transportation in Downers Grove, Illinois, had a habit of consistently misusing words. Her speech displayed classic examples of malapropism, which is a humorous misuse of the English language, using words that sound similar to the correct one but ridiculously wrong in context. The word "malapropism" is based on a character in a play, Mrs. Malaprop (R.B. Sheridan's comedy <u>THE RIVALS</u>), who was noted for her misuse of words. My co-worker would say things such as, "neon stockings" instead of "nylon stockings," "fire distinguisher" instead of "fire extinguisher", or "it's just a pigment of your imagination" instead of "a figment of your imagination."

She always took me by surprise. It would take me a moment to realize she had used the wrong word. I never corrected her nor let her know how humorous it was. I always wished that I had written them all down because they were delightfully entertaining.

We misuse words as well, but some words we misuse are not as humorous. We sometimes say "yes" when we should say "no". Titus 2:11-12 tells us, *"For the grace of God...teaches us to say 'No' to ungodliness and worldly passions, and to live self-controlled, upright and godly lives in this present age."* Many times we say "no" when we should say "yes." Jesus asked Peter in John 21:14, *"...do you truly love me more than these?"*

There are times we say "can't" instead of "can." Philippians 4:13 tells us, *"I can do everything through him who gives me strength."* We may say "tomorrow" when we should say "today." *"For as long as it's still God's today, keep each other on your toes so sin doesn't slow down your reflexes."* (Hebrews 3:13)

It is also possible that we say "mine" when we should say "yours." 1 Corinthians 6:19 says, *"Do you not know that your body is a temple of the Holy Spirit, who is in you, whom you have received from God? You are not your own."* We belong to God.

Words are important. They are not just verbal sounds. They are powerful tools and the small words are just as powerful as the big ones. We have thousands of words to choose from each day and those choices shape our destiny. If we talk with someone long enough, we usually find out what he or she truly believes because what is said stems from our hearts. Matthew 12:34 tells us that *"out of the overflow of the heart, the mouth speaks."*

We would be wise to choose our words carefully and be cautious of the constant inner dialogue we hold within ourselves. They can be statements of criticism or praise, truth or lies, doubt or faith. Every word matters! Words can change our lives. *"May the words of my mouth and the meditation of my heart be pleasing in your sight, O Lord, my Rock and my Redeemer."* (Psalm 19:14) What did you say?

> O my Father God, I stand in awe of your goodness. I see your footprints everywhere. They are within me. When I turn within, I am on holy ground, for your presence is in every flaming bush of emotion, in every call that comes from the deeps of my being. I am your Temple. May everything within your temple say, "Glory!"  ~ E. Stanley Jones (1884–1973)

**FOOD FOR THOUGHT**

~ When is the last time I said "yes" when I should have said "no"?

~ Is my inner dialog with myself encouraging or discouraging?

~ In what ways do my words shape my destiny?

# A RAINBOW WANNABE

When our son, Bruce, was four months old, I took him to the pediatrician for a check-up. The doctor looked me in the eye and said, "Your son doesn't like his green veggies, does he!" It surprised me that the color of my baby's skin would reveal his preference for creamed carrots and squash over green beans and spinach!

If the food that goes inside us affects the color of our skin, it is safe to assume that our spiritual diet affects the color of our spirit. If we fill our hearts and minds with the things of this world, the color of our spirit will suffer. If we feast on God's Word and spend time in His presence, our spirit will glow with the vibrant colors of spiritual health.

I was in a discussion group one time at church when the leader asked the question, "What color are you spiritually?" One participant said she was definitely blue, representing depression, because of all the recent failures in her life. One said her spirit was yellow, representing sunshine and the warmth of God's love and forgiveness. Another said she was plaid, because she was a little bit of everything, but having difficulty finding God's perfect will for her life. My young friend, Sarah, loves vibrant colors. When I asked her that question, she said her spirit was green to represent spiritual growth, but that she is a "neon-green wannabe." In other words, she wanted to glow with spiritual health.

How important is color? Research reveals that color affects us in many ways. Some colors give us energy and make us more creative. Some colors are soothing and relaxing. There is no one color that is more important than the others. We need them all.

Our daughter, Kerry, is an artist and loves all colors. She says,

As an artist I am constantly aware of light, color, forms and imagery. These things take on a spiritual side to me and sharpen or concentrate my awareness of God's handiwork. Color assails me continually. I see the colors in the world swirling about me. Everywhere there is color, there is energy - serene greens, yellows, reds and browns flickering in the light and wind in the many forms of nature - pulsing streams of colors flowing with crowds of people. They fill me to the point of overflowing onto my canvas.

God gave us the gift of color. God's promise to Noah came in the form of a colorful rainbow. *"I have set my rainbow in the clouds, and it will be the sign of the covenant between me and the earth."* (Genesis 9:13) God chose the rainbow as a symbol of hope.

What color are we spiritually? We all have areas that have lost their luster. What color do we want to be? Do we want all God has for us or are we tempted to settle for a faded relationship?

Are we "rainbow wannabes"? Are we ready to fill our spirits with the vibrant colors of faith, bursting with energy and glowing with health? The rainbow is a symbol of hope that we can be (both physically and spiritually) all God wants us to be.

> O Christ, our Morning Star, Splendor of Light Eternal, shining with the glory of the rainbow, come and waken us from the greyness of our apathy, and renew in us your gift of hope.
> ~ Bede the Venerable (672-735)

**FOOD FOR THOUGHT**

~ What color am I spiritually?

~ In what ways am I inspired by color?

~ How does the Word of God awaken me from the greyness of my apathy?

# CAUGHT OFF GUARD

When our daughter, Rhonda, was attending Northern Illinois University, I went to the college one night to join her and her college friends for dinner and a movie. (Allow me to give you some advice. Never let college students pick the movie!) We went to see "Death Trap" with Michael Caine and Christopher Reeve. Partway through the movie, everyone breathed a sigh of relief when the evil man was killed and buried in the backyard. A short time later, however, he came crashing abruptly through a window, alive and well and as evil as ever. Rhonda and her friends were greatly amused at my reaction to the window crashing scene because I nearly jumped out of my chair. I was relaxed and totally unprepared for the sudden turn of events. I was "caught off guard."

Life is like that sometimes. Everything is going well and we assume everything will continue to go well. When life delivers a sudden blow, our reactions are usually less than constructive. In the Bible, when Moses returned from speaking with God on the mountain, he carried in his hands the 10 commandments written by the finger of God. When he saw the people worshiping the golden calf, he was suddenly angered and smashed the stone tablets on the ground. He was "caught off guard."

Eve was caught off guard when she listened to the lies of Satan. Adam was caught off guard when Eve offered him a taste of innocent looking fruit. Lot's wife was caught off guard because she didn't believe God meant what He said. Samson was said to have superhuman strength, yet he was caught off guard by one deceptive female named Delilah. King David was caught off guard by the beauty of Bathsheba. Judas Iscariot was caught off guard because he valued earthly riches more than heavenly riches.

If the Bible characters were caught off guard so easily, rest assured that we are not immune. The Bible tells us that we can learn from

their mistakes. *"These things happened to them as examples and were written down as warnings for us...So, if you think you are standing firm, be careful that you don't fall!"*
(1 Corinthians 10:11-12)

When we least expect it, life can explode and we are likely to say and do things we will regret later. This includes ways in which we sabotage our own bodies. When we are unprepared for the stressful times, we gravitate to unhealthy foods that we believe will help us feel better.

Evil is NEVER buried and gone. It has a way of resurrecting and crashing into our lives when we least expect it. During stressful times, our emotions overwhelm us and we do not make thoughtful, wise decisions. Although we know stressful times will come, we don't always know when or where. How do we prepare? Jesus tells us to, *"Watch and pray so that you will not fall into temptation. The spirit is willing, but the flesh is weak."* (Matthew 26:41) Both watching and praying will protect us from being "caught off guard!"

---
Divine Chemist, you have hidden in the heart of food the germs of vitality and health - we thank you for this. Help us now to hunt them out and utilize them to the full. For they are your gift.
~ E. Stanley Jones (1884–1973)

---

**FOOD FOR THOUGHT**

~ When is the last time something caught me off guard?

~ When the Bible tells me to "watch and pray," what does it mean to watch?

~ Do I think I am standing firm? Am I?

## DANGER! DANGER!

My husband's job took him on many overseas business trips. On one of Jack's trips to Tanzania, Africa, their group scheduled a guided safari to the Serengeti, a national park of rolling plains covering 5,700 square miles. It is estimated that some three million large animals call the Serengeti home. He shares the following story.

   During our guided safari, we had to come to a complete stop to wait for an elephant to get off the road. At another spot along the road, we had to slow down as a giraffe was sauntering down the road in front of us. The guide was determined to find some lions for us, but to no avail. On the way to the supposed lion habitat, we stopped at another small lagoon where some hippos were bathing. When hippos bathe, about all one can see above the water are two ears, two eyes and two nostrils. The hippos were on the other side of the lagoon, so I decided to walk around to the other side to get some close-up pictures. I was standing about three feet from the edge of the water with tall grass between me and the water's edge.

   I was busily taking my photos when our guide came running down the path toward me shouting, "Danger, danger, crocodile! Danger! Crocodile!" He grabbed me by the arm and quickly pulled me away. At the same time, we heard a splash and saw Mr. Crocodile slip into the water. From a distance, our guide and the rest of the group had seen him resting in the tall grass at my feet, but I was completely unaware of his presence.

My husband's trip to Tanzania was during the time the movie, "Crocodile Dundee" was popular in the theaters. So our children made a large sign for the front yard to welcome him home that read, "Welcome home, Crocodile Dad-dee!"

When my husband stood near the tall grass by the edge of the water, he was completely unaware of the nearby danger. The only thought that occupied his mind was the pleasure of being able to share some great photographs of hippos with family and friends. We, too, are not always aware of the dangers that come as a result of our unhealthy eating habits. Our minds are focused on the pleasures of taste and satisfaction.

2 Timothy 3:1-4 tells us that in the last days, among other things, *"people will be lovers of themselves, lovers of money"* and *"lovers of pleasure rather than lovers of God."* With the decline in the economy, church giving has seen a dramatic decrease. And yet people are eating out more than ever and spend annually over $25 billion on video games, hardware and accessories, over $70 billion dollars for carbonated soft drinks and almost $30 billion dollars on candy.

Focusing on pleasure can be dangerous. Jesus calls out to us, "Danger! Danger!" and tries to pull us away. Our job is to listen and yield to His direction.

> Lord, Your servant, the Apostle Paul, was in danger from rivers, in danger from bandits, in danger from his own countrymen, in danger from Gentiles, in danger in the city, in danger in the country, in danger at sea, and in danger from false brothers. Yet your power was made perfect in his weakness. Help me to know that your grace is sufficient for me as well.
> ~ based on 2 Corinthians 12:8-10

FOOD FOR THOUGHT

~ When is the last time I used scripture to defeat Satan?

~ When would Satan consider it an opportune time to temp me?

~ Can we hear the call of "danger" or is the music of the world too loud?

# TRUST

When our granddaughter, Christine, was three years old, she had a game she loved to play. When we would go shopping and arrive at a store, she always pretended to be asleep in her car seat.

One particular day, when we arrived in the Walmart parking lot, I endeavored to get her out of her car seat although she was feigning sleep. I knew it was part of the game, so I played along. She permitted me to get her unbuckled and stand her on her feet, but continued to "sleep-walk" through the parking lot to the store. She took my hand and allowed me to lead her all the way while holding her eyes tightly closed, tilting her head to rest on her shoulder, and all the while displaying a smirk on her tiny face.

I'm sure passers-by were speculating to themselves, "I wonder what's wrong with that poor child?" It was hilarious. I finally laughed hard enough that she began to laugh too. She was pleased as punch with herself because she thought she had made a pretty good joke. The amazing part was the fact that she trusted me completely. She didn't peek once. She just closed her eyes tightly and went wherever I led her.

What a blessing it would be if we could trust God just as completely as Christine trusted me, putting our hand in His and allowing Him to lead us wherever He pleases. It wouldn't matter how many rocks were in the road, He would lead us safely to our destination.

Some of us have had some pretty rocky pathways lately. There have been financial difficulties and serious illnesses and strained relationships. And we have been tripping over our own rocks of self-centeredness and self-indulgence.

We can trust God to lead us! He is the Good Shepherd. Psalm 23:1 says, *"The Lord is my Shepherd, I shall not be in want."* Just as a shepherd leads his sheep to green pastures and quiet waters, our Good Shepherd leads us to abundance and peace. He knows what is best for us. When we do not follow His lead and insist on our own way, not only do we put ourselves in danger, but we sacrifice any hope of true satisfaction. The problem is more than our lack of wisdom and skill. The problem is our blindness. We don't know where we are going.

God said in Isaiah 42:16, *"I will lead the blind by ways they have not known, along unfamiliar paths I will guide them; I will turn the darkness into light before them and make the rough places smooth. These are the things I will do; I will not forsake them."*

Yes, we can "trust" God! He will never forsake us. When our souls are saturated with the knowledge of His unlimited wisdom and power and our hearts rest in the assurance that our Great Shepherd is rich in mercy and love, we will be more than happy to follow His lead!

> You, O LORD, keep my lamp burning; my God turns my darkness into light. With your help I can advance against a troop; with my God I can scale a wall. ~ Psalm 18:28, 29

**FOOD FOR THOUGHT**

~ Do I trust God 100% of the time? 80%? 60%?

~ What rocks of life am I tripping over?

~ If God has unlimited wisdom and power and He loves me, why do I worry?

# RECIPE FOR DISASTER

A missionary from Mexico was visiting our church in Newberry, Michigan. My husband and I, who were youth directors at the time, thought it would be a great idea to invite her to our home for dinner, along with the entire youth group, for an authentic Mexican meal. When having company, it's usually best to stay with tried and true recipes that have worked well in the past, but since I wanted a "real" Mexican meal, I went to the Library and copied some recipes out of a Mexican cookbook. My husband warned me that I should cut down on the hot sauce because most of our guests were not accustomed to eating spicy foods but, since I wanted it to be "authentic," I ignored his request.

You guessed it. The entire youth group missed school the next day with intestinal problems. My husband and I were sick as well. We never found out if the missionary was sick. We were afraid to ask.

Another time when I was having friends over for dinner, I decided to make a pork stir-fry, something I was confident I could do well. The problem surfaced because the bottle of soy sauce and the bottle of Mexican vanilla were almost identical in appearance. Yes, you are right again. I grabbed the Mexican vanilla for my stir fry instead of the soy sauce. In addition to being almost inedible, it was rather embarrassing.

You may enjoy a good chuckle at my expense, but we may as well admit that all of us have probably used a "recipe for disaster" at one time or another. Sometimes we are so anxious to impress or overconfident that we forget what is important. If we are so anxious to give company our best, we should, all the more, desire to give God our best! In the old testament, God demanded that the sacrifices brought to Him be without defect. "'*When you bring injured, crippled or diseased animals and offer them as sacrifices, should I accept them from your hands?' says the LORD.*" (Malachi

1:13) God does not want our second best and He doesn't want our leftovers.

The best gift we can give God is the gift of ourselves. *"Do your best to present yourself to God as one approved, a workman who does not need to be ashamed and who correctly handles the word of truth."* (2 Timothy 2:15) We believe in excellence. If we purchase a house or choose a school system for our children or search for a surgeon for a needed operation, we want the best. When we give to God, we sometimes settle for "good enough." To give the gift of ourselves, it must be the best self we can give, both physically and spiritually, to enable us to serve wherever He leads.

In His Holy Word, God lays out His recipe for a sanctified life that will please Him. When we use ingredients of questionable quality or carelessly alter life's recipe to suit ourselves, it is always a "recipe for disaster!"

---

Forgive me my sins, O Lord, forgive me the sins of my youth and the sins of my age, the sins of my soul, and the sins of my body, my secret and my whispering sins, my presumptuous and my crying sins, the sins that I have done to please myself, and the sins that I have done to please others. Forgive me those sins which I know and those sins which I know not; forgive them, O Lord, forgive them all of your great goodness.
~ Private Devotions (1560)

---

**FOOD FOR THOUGHT**

~ Who am I most anxious to please…people or God?

~ In what way do I alter God's recipe for a sanctified life to please myself?

~ How do I offer my body as a living sacrifice?

# IT'S ALL ABOUT BALANCE

Our grandsons, Ben and Brad, ride unicycles. In 2002, after having the unicycles for less than two years, they won some awards in the International Unicycle World Championship competition in Seattle. In 2003, both boys won awards in the National Unicycling Championships in Minneapolis. Ben was the intermediate class-A artistic freestyle national champion and Brad was the overall racing national champion of the 9-10 year old age group. My son, Bruce, also rides a unicycle. He shares his own claim to fame in Minneapolis: "I competed in the one-mile, off-road unicycle course. I did not get last place because I beat two six-year-old girls who got lost in the woods."

Bruce started a unicycle club in their neighborhood. He called it The Unicycle Uni-Versity. About fifty kids and adults participated and Bruce owned twenty-six unicycles which he rented to the members. There is something intriguing about a unicycle: riding is all about balance. Unicyclists have to balance their whole body or they will fall. A healthy lifestyle is also about balance, balancing the desires of the flesh with the desires of the spirit. If we get off-balance, we could end up with spiritual skinned knees, or worse, with a spiritual concussion. Sometimes we try to adapt all our human desires and fit them into a spiritual mold. But God gave us both – a body and a spirit. He gave us hunger signals to tell us when we are hungry and He gave us taste buds to enjoy our food.

Unicycling gives freedom. In unicycling, as opposed to bicycling, the legs and the balance of the body do *all* of the work, leaving the arms free to fly in the wind. Finding a good balance between the body's desires and the spirit's desires gives us the freedom to enjoy life to the fullest. If we are hungry, it is a good thing to give in to that hunger and eat. Much of our hunger, however, is not "body" hunger, but "head" hunger. Giving in to head hunger will throw us off balance. If we want our spiritual desires to develop to their full potential, we have to treat our bodies with respect.

There are some dieting philosophies that would teach us to picture our food crawling with worms and maggots in order to make us feel disgusted with food and not want to eat it. My philosophy is just the opposite: eat and be thankful. Choose a wholesome food and concentrate on the wonderful flavors and textures. We all know what wonderful attributes foods have – some cold and crisp and crunchy – some warm and filling and some with smells almost too wonderful to imagine. Taste buds are God's idea. He did not create taste buds to torture us; I'm convinced He gave us taste buds because He loves us. Most of the time, we have ruined the abilities of our taste buds with too much salt, sugar, grease, and artificial additives, making us unable to enjoy wholesome foods that are not "doctored up."

It's all about balance. God wants things to be in balance - both in our personal lives and in our spiritual lives. *"For God is not a God of disorder but of peace."* (1 Corinthians 14:33) That is our goal – to balance the body and the spirit, striving to satisfy the desires of each using only God's best!

> O Lord, who loves all men, cause the light of your unchangeable wisdom to shine into our hearts, and open the eyes of our minds to the understanding of all your revealed truth. Put into us the fear of your blessed commandments, that by subduing all fleshly lusts, we may make progress in spiritual life, both thinking and acting in all things according to your good pleasure.
> ~ Henry Drummond (1851-1897)

**FOOD FOR THOUGHT**

~ Are my body and spirit in balance?

~ How much do I appreciate the food I eat?

~ How do I tell the difference between body hunger and head hunger?

# ADDICTED TO MEDIOCRITY

My sister-in-law, Ginger, was cooking pizza for us during our visit to her home in Payson, Arizona. Although she set the oven to the required temperature and for the required amount of time, the pizzas were doughy and undercooked when she took them out of the oven. Maybe her oven had a variance, or maybe it was because she was cooking two pizzas at once. I have also read that at altitudes over 3000 feet, baked goods may need adjustments in time or temperature and we were at 5000 feet. Whatever the cause, she made the wise decision to put them back into the oven a little longer. When she took the pizzas out the second time, they were perfect.

There is a scripture in Hosea 7:8 that says, "...*Ephraim* (one of the tribes of Israel) *is a flat cake not turned over.*" I'm not sure exactly what God is trying to say in this scripture, but I imagine it means that the people of Ephraim were a little "half-baked" like our pizzas. Perhaps they did not spend enough time in the warmth of God's love to allow the finishing touches of His grace to complete their spiritual growth.

Some of us may qualify as half-baked Christians. We have just enough religion to make us miserable. I saw a book one time and, although I have not read it, I thought the title was intriguing. It was called, "Addicted to Mediocrity." Is it true? Are we content with less than God's best? Do we stray from God's plans for our lives because it seems like too much effort?

Not one of us would like to be known as a mediocre person, yet how often do we pursue excellence or display the stamina and perseverance necessary to give God our best. God was very specific in His instructions to the Israelites: sacrifices to Him were to be "without defect." The Israelites were to give Him only the best.

Often, we do not pursue excellence in our weight-loss efforts either. Some of us are half-baked dieters. We are addicted to mediocrity: we are satisfied and pleased with ourselves that we made a tiny bit of effort, and that we are not as overweight as the lady we saw at a restaurant last week. We start each diet with great enthusiasm, but never finish. We begin an exercise program but it only lasts a week or so. We are lulled into complacency about the future, fanaticizing that someday, somehow, we will surely reach our goal.

If we are half-baked in any area, there are only two things that will finish the baking - time and temperature. Spending time in God's presence in the warmth of His love will break our inclination to be "addicted to mediocrity." We will not be happy until we make every effort to do the things that please our Heavenly Father.

Hebrews 12:12-13 tells us: *"Don't sit around on your hands! No more dragging your feet! Clear the path for long-distance runners so no one will trip and fall, so no one will step in a hole and sprain an ankle. Help each other out. And run for it!"* (The Message.) There's nothing "mediocre" about that!

> We love you, O our God; and we desire to love you more and more. Give us love, sweetest of all gifts, which knows no enemy. O most loving Father of Jesus Christ, from whom flows all love, let our hearts, frozen in sin, cold to you and cold to others, be warmed by this divine fire. ~ Prayer of Anselm (12th Century)

**FOOD FOR THOUGHT**

~ How often do I pursue excellence?

~ In what areas do I have a tendency to be half-baked?

~ How do I master the habit of finishing what I start?

# THE GIFT OF FREEDOM

I had a great deal of freedom when I was eleven. In fact, I had entirely too much freedom! My mother could not afford a babysitter during the summer so the neighbors were supposed to keep a watchful eye on me. Although it was a safer world in 1951, my friends and I were never lacking in imagination for exciting but risky adventures. We loved playing on the railroad tracks or climbing over the fence at the junk yard to find "good" junk.

One day, my four friends and I were feeling especially brave and adventurous. We decided to hitchhike from our town of Aurora, Illinois to Naperville, Illinois. We were first picked up by a lonely elderly lady who talked for the whole trip and wished us well on our journey before she dropped us off. We played for a while down by the river. One of my friends fell in the water. We pooled our money to buy her a pair of shorts and hoped her jeans would be dry before she arrived home so that her parents would not find out what happened.

On the way home we were picked up by a young man. One of my friends bravely sat in the front and the rest of us all crammed into the back seat. We naively felt very smug and safe because one girl had a jackknife in her pocket. We arrived home safely with no clue of the enormous risk we had just taken. To our chagrin, one of my friends felt guilty and confessed to her parents, getting us all into big trouble.

It goes without saying that five innocent young girls should not have been hitchhiking with strangers. I am extremely grateful we did not end up as a tragic statistic. Yes, as a child I had a great deal of freedom, but through the misuse of that freedom, I put myself and others in great danger. As we grow older and more mature, it should mean that we will have the strength and ability to handle our freedom more wisely. Unfortunately, that is not always the case.

Today, the society in which we live offers each of us a great deal of freedom. From the selection of careers to the decision of which television programs to watch or even to the foods we eat, we are bombarded with choices. How we handle those choices can drastically interfere with the purposes to which God has called us. We must remember that "Emancipation from the bondage of the soil is no freedom for the tree." (Rabindranath Tagore)

Certain restrictions exist for a purpose and by honoring them, we are richly rewarded. May God give us the wisdom to know which restrictions should be honored and which should be challenged. *"I pray that you may have the power to comprehend, with all the saints, what is the breadth and length and height and depth, and to know the love of Christ that surpasses knowledge, so that you may be filled with all the fullness of God."* (Ephesians 3:18-19)

God has gifted us with freedom. We are truly free to be ourselves, but if we want optimal results, we are only free to be the persons God intended.

> O God, my spiritual and corporal existence is yours since you are my Creator. But my will is mine because you have created it as free and want it to remain such. However, I am free to offer it in homage to you and to make it a sacrifice of praise and honor to you. Hence, I give my will entirely to you, so that it no longer belongs to me.  ~ St. Louise de Marillac (1591-1660)

**FOOD FOR THOUGHT**

~ How do I mishandle the freedoms God has given me?

~ What responsibilities come with freedom?

~ In what ways could it be dangerous to be free of God's restrictions?

## CUT OUT THE NOISE!

One night, around 3:00 a.m., my husband and I were awakened by strange sounds coming from the kitchen. We listened closely and heard voices. My husband bravely ventured out to the kitchen and found that the television was playing. It had apparently come on all by itself. He turned it off and went back to bed. This has happened several times since then at various hours. We have no idea how or why it happens, but it is strangely unsettling to hear voices in our house in the middle of the night.

There are a lot of sounds in this world - some welcome and some not. We first have to decide how to define the word, "sound." A sound is an energy transmitted by waves through a material, such as air, and upon reaching the ear, we can hear. The age old question still exists, "If a tree falls in the woods and no one is there to hear it, does it make any sound?"

Some sounds are classified as noise, which is a sound that is noticeably unpleasant or one that does not seem to belong to its source. The classification of something as a sound or a noise may depend on the personality, age or background of the person listening to it. "Elevator music" can be very soothing to a 90-year-old and at the same time extremely irritating to a 15-year-old. Rock music could also produce some contrasting reactions. To a busy executive with no children, the sound of a small baby's cry might be irritating, but to the young mother who just gave birth, it is the sweetest sound on earth. To someone who works at night and sleeps during the daytime, the sound of small children laughing and playing outside the window would be unwelcome, but to the grandparents who adore them, it is a sweet and joyful sound.

What is noise to God? Our prayers would *never* fit into that category. God loves to hear our prayers. They are welcome sounds to His ears. Jeremiah 29:12 says, "*Then you will call upon me and come and pray to me, and I will listen to you."* What God *does* consider "noise" is our griping and complaining. Numbers 11:1 tells us, *"Now the people complained about their hardships in the hearing of the LORD, and when he heard them his anger was aroused..."* Philippians 2:14 tells us to..."*Do ALL things without grumbling...*" "All things" includes giving up the excess food that is detrimental to our health and doing sufficient exercise to make our bodies healthy. How many times do we start a new diet or health plan and find ourselves griping and complaining about how difficult it is?

In reality, developing an "attitude of gratitude" is necessary for the success of our efforts. When we stop complaining and begin to appreciate all our gifts from God, our desire for excess food will begin to diminish and we will consider it a privilege to care for the wonderful bodies God has given us. So let's stop our griping and complaining. Let's "cut out the noise!"

> Almighty God, Father of all mercies, we give you humble thanks for all your goodness and loving-kindness to us. And, we pray, give us such an awareness of your mercies, that with truly thankful hearts we may show forth your praise, not only with our lips, but in our lives, by giving up ourselves to your service, and by walking before you in holiness and righteousness all our days.
> ~ Book of Common Prayer (1549)

## FOOD FOR THOUGHT

~ Do I do ALL things without grumbling?

~ How can I best develop an "attitude of gratitude"?

~ In what ways does a grateful heart benefit my health?

# CRABBY

When we lived in Maryland, we loved to go crabbing for Maryland Blue Crabs in the Chesapeake Bay. Our children enjoyed catching crabs the old-fashioned way by dangling a raw chicken neck on a string into the water. When they felt a tug on the string, they would use a long-handled pole with a landing net to scoop up the crab. The trick was getting the crab into the pail. To the inexperienced, it would seem like a simple matter to scoop up the crab with the net, turn the net upside down over the bucket and dump it out. Crabs, however, always seem to be a little crabby. They have minds of their own and have no intention of landing in our bucket, using their claws to clamp tightly onto the net.

We used tongs to try prying the claws loose. Sometimes it worked, sometimes it did not. If we made the mistake of holding the net too closely to the edge of the bucket, the crab would quickly drop and scramble over the side, scurrying sideways across the boardwalk and plunging into the bay to freedom. Our barefooted children would scream and dance, keeping their toes out of harm's way until the crab was in the water.

We tempted the crabs with a nice fresh bucket of water. Some crabs got tired of holding on, relaxed their grip and dropped into our pail. Others were stubborn enough to keep holding on and it seemed impossible to pry them loose. They tenaciously waited and watched for their opportunity to escape to freedom. Our little crabs had every reason to be crabby - we were trying to take them captive. We were not only taking away their freedom, but also threatening their lives.

We are in danger of being taken captive as well, by Satan. We need to hold on tightly because our very lives are being threatened. He entices us to relax and loosen our grip on our resolve not to sin. The Bible tells us: *"Be self-controlled and alert. Your enemy, the devil, prowls around like a roaring lion looking for someone to devour."* (1 Peter 5:8) The real problem is that he doesn't look like a lion. 2 Corinthians 11:13 tells us that, *"Satan himself masquerades as an angel of light."* Some of our little crabs were smart enough to know that the enticing bucket of fresh water below them was a trap and not at all equal to swimming free in the bay. It pays to be a little crabby when it comes to temptation. We must not take the dangers lightly. Sometimes we tire of holding on to what we know is true, relax our grip and succumb to the lure of the immediate.

If we do not want to be defeated, we can choose to be victorious. The Bible tells us: *"...Resist the devil, and he will flee from you."* (James 4:7) Jesus was just a little crabby in his response to the temptations of Satan. He quoted scripture and simply said, *"...Beat it, Satan!..."* (Matthew 4:10 - MSG) It's time for us to get "crabby" with the devil!

> Give us, O Lord, a steadfast heart, which no unworthy affection may drag downwards; give us an unconquered heart, which no unworthy purpose may tempt aside. Bestow upon us also, O Lord our God, understanding to know you, diligence to seek you, wisdom to find you and a faithfulness that may finally embrace you; through Jesus Christ our Lord.
> ~ St. Thomas Aquinas (1225-1274)

**FOOD FOR THOUGHT**

~ Am I less tolerant of other people's sins than I am of my own?

~ How alluring is a fresh bucket of instant gratification?

~ What is the best way to inform Satan that my resolve cannot and will not be broken?

# LAUGHTER, THE BEST MEDICINE

There is nothing more refreshing than the sound of laughter. I love it when my grandchildren get the giggles; the sound makes the whole house come alive. We had an experience one time at Michigamme United Methodist Family Camp that gave our family a good laugh.

On Thursday evening at camp, the log chapel is set up for communion. After a brief service in the dining hall, we were invited to go to the chapel, one family at a time, to take communion together as a family. When our turn came, we entered the chapel and seated ourselves on the wooden folding chairs with my husband, Jack, at the head of the table. As my husband sat down, we heard a loud crack as the chair collapsed. He quietly and reverently set the broken chair aside, replacing it with another one, but as soon as he sat down, the second chair broke as well. This time (not so reverently), amid snickers from the family, he again replaced the chair. When the third chair broke, the atmosphere was anything but reverent. The family was doubled over with laughter. Although the fourth chair held, we were sure we heard God laughing as well. The humor continued into the following year when someone called out, "Hide the chairs, Jack's here!" as we arrived.

The multiple problems we face every day have a tendency to make us serious-minded, but we need laughter. Jesus wanted us to have joy. *"I have told you this so that my joy may be in you and that your joy may be complete."* (John 15:11) Part of the reason we struggle so much with self-control is that we are stressed and depressed and have lost our ability to see the joy and wonder of every day life. Joy is elusive if our focus is on our problems instead of on God. How many of us could write joyful words from a jail cell like the Apostle Paul did: *"Rejoice in the Lord always. I will say it again: Rejoice!"* (Philippians 4:5)

In 1907, Henry van Dyke wrote the poem "Joyful, Joyful We Adore Thee" which was later set to music and is still being sung in churches today. The words to this hymn continue to inspire us and remind us that laughter and joy are possible in the problem-filled world in which we live.

> Joyful, joyful, we adore Thee,
> God of glory, Lord of love;
> Hearts unfold like flowers before Thee,
> Opening to the sun above.
> Melt the clouds of sin and sadness;
> Drive the dark of doubt away;
> Giver of immortal gladness,
> Fill us with the light of day!

Yes, laughter is the best medicine! It triggers the release of endorphins, which are natural feel-good chemicals, giving us a sense of well-being. The gift of laughter is truly one of God's greatest gifts.

> LORD, you are my Lord; apart from you I have no good thing. You have made known to me the path of life; you will fill me with joy in your presence, with eternal pleasures at your right hand.
> ~ Psalm 16:1,11

**FOOD FOR THOUGHT**

~ When is the last time I discovered joy and wonder in an everyday event?

~ How does stress weaken my self-control?

~ Is joy a choice? Why or why not?

## THE BEST LAID PLANS

My friend, Janie Shoemaker, returned from vacation and shared this story:

Just returned from an interesting vacation in Panama City Beach, Florida. No sunshine since we left Southern Illinois on Wednesday. HUGE waves (double red flags on ocean - not allowed in). Tropical Storm Lee really is messing up fun time in the ocean. STILL, most interesting trip ever!! Hubby, daughter, grandson, granddaughter helped rescue a lady who was riding a motorized wheelchair made for the beach and it quit on her. Tide was coming in and waves washing up to her chair. 911 was called but they said it wasn't their problem. MY family took a chair from the pool area at our condo, her hubby moved her over to it (she was paralyzed from waist down) and they carried her up to the roadside. That was three days ago - chair still sitting on the beach covered with sand from incoming tides.

Then yesterday on our way home, we were first on the scene of an accident with two young ladies and three small children. She flipped the car three times and was upside down in ditch. We got the kids in the car with us and called 911. Ambulances and police arrived and transported them all to the hospital. Sure hope they're all o.k. We went through heavy rain all the way home until Paducah. I'm so glad to be home safe and sound. It was not a beach type weekend but STILL very interesting!

We make a lot of plans in this life. It's good to plan. It's necessary to plan, but sometimes no matter how carefully we plan, things go differently. For example, the lady in the wheelchair most likely planned on a leisurely ride on the beach to enjoy God's creation of sun, water and sky. When she ran into a problem, she probably planned on getting help from 911, but her help came from an unexpected source - tourists who were willing to put aside their own plans to help someone in need. The two ladies with small children certainly did not plan to be in an automobile accident. No one planned on Tropical Storm Lee creating havoc on people and property. Janie and her family originally planned on a fun-filled, sun-soaked vacation on the beach, but God planned for them to be in the right place at the right time so that they could be of service to others. Although their original plans were interrupted, they came home strangely fulfilled in a different way.

God intends for us to find enjoyment in living, but we need to remember that the joy that comes from serving others has the capability of surpassing all other pleasures. Everything we do, even if it is just cooking and cleaning, can be done for the love of Him who loved us first. We should not be surprised if God interrupts our "best laid plans" for pleasure and gives us an opportunity to serve others. *"Sitting down, Jesus...said, 'If anyone wants to be first, he must be the very last, and the servant of all.'"* (Mark 9:35)

> O Lord of pots and pans and things, since I have no time to be
> A great saint by doing lovely things, or watching late with Thee,
> Or dreaming in the dawn light, or storming Heaven's gates,
> Make me a saint by getting meals, and washing up the plates.
> Warm all the kitchen with Thy love and light it with Thy peace;
> Forgive me all my worrying and make my grumbling cease.
> Thou who loved to give men food in room or by the sea,
> Accept the service that I do - I do it unto Thee.
> ~ Brother Lawrence (1614-1691)

## FOOD FOR THOUGHT

~ Am I a planner? How upset do I get when my plans fall apart?

~ In what way is the joy of serving others more satisfying than pleasing myself?

~ Why is serving others sometimes called an "opportunity"?

# DECONTAMINATION

Shortly after we moved to Las Vegas, Nevada in 1988, there was a major explosion at Pepcon, an ammonium perchlorate processing plant to the south of town. Both my husband and I heard the noise and rushed outside to see the plume of smoke rising in the air. Although the plant was five miles from our house, our front door and an upstairs window were damaged.

The Pepcon disaster claimed two lives and injured 372 people. Ammonium perchlorate is used as an oxidizer in space vehicles and is highly volatile. The explosion was massive because there was an estimated 4000 tons of the product stored at the site and there was a high-pressure natural gas line running underneath the plant which ruptured during one of the explosions. A total of seven explosions caused close to $100 million in damages. The largest explosion measured 3.5 on the Richter scale.

Since my husband worked for the Office of Pipeline Safety for the State of Nevada, he was called to investigate the accident. He says:

> The explosion created a cavern and ripped up a 16-inch natural gas line going through the property. I spent most of my first summer out in the desert at the site. I've never drunk so much Gatorade in my life. Adjacent to this facility was a Kidd marshmallow plant that was also completely leveled. Do you know, marshmallows do not come out the best during an explosion. What a sticky gooey mess all over the place!
>
> Until the atmosphere was deemed clear, we had to wear the traditional white "monkey suits" used for entering contaminated areas. Naturally, these suits are designed so air will not penetrate them. At the end of the period in the contaminated atmosphere, we would clear the quarantined area and stand in a kid's inflatable wading pool to be hosed down. Then we would

remove our boots and pour about a quart of perspiration out of each boot. This was tough work for a north-woodsman like me who cannot take hot weather.

Because of my husband's intimate contact with dangerous residue, he had to be decontaminated after each visit. We are in close contact every day with some of the undesirable values of this world. There is residue left in our lives from immoral television and movies and self-pampering magazine articles. There is increased crime in every level from the street gangs to some of our politicians. All of these things contaminate our spiritual lives. We must put ourselves through a decontamination process to remove all possible danger to our soul. It's best to avoid the residue if we can, but when we are compelled to have contact, we must take time to cleanse ourselves of worldly impurities by spending time in God's presence.

Although it will be tough work, let the "decontamination" process begin. *"Since we have these promises, dear friends, let us purify ourselves from everything that contaminates body and spirit, perfecting holiness out of reverence for God."* (2 Corinthians 7:1)

---
Thank you, Jesus, that your blood purifies me from all sin. You have promised that if I confess my sin, you are faithful and just and will forgive my sin and purify me from all unrighteousness.
~ based on 1 John 1:7,9

---

**FOOD FOR THOUGHT**

~ How do I decide which values of the world are undesirable?

~ What can I do to limit contact with dangerous worldly values?

~ What does the spiritual purification process include?

# REMEMBER WHO YOU ARE

The Bible tells us, "*A good name is more desirable than great riches...*" (Proverbs 22:1) As a young child, I hated my name. I was named after my grandmother, Idella Pearl Chapin. My maiden name, Idella Liskey, gave the other children ample ammunition to make fun of me. I was a shy kid and the barbs stung. They would taunt me on a regular basis with chants such as, "Idella Liskey loves to drink whiskey," or "Ideller has a feller in the cellar." Kids can be cruel.

As I matured, I began to love having a unique name. I have met only a small number of people in my lifetime with the same first name as mine. One time, by coincidence, I happened to sit next to a lady on an airplane whose name was Idella.

Names are important. We always knew we were in trouble when our mother called us by our full names. Husbands and wives usually have pet names for each other such as "honey," "sweetheart" or even "my little turtle dove." Sometimes we have pet nicknames for our children. My father used to call me "Bedo" but I never knew where the name came from. My daughter called our grandson Samuel "Bambino," the Italian name for "little boy." Later it became "Sambeeno" and eventually ended up as "Beeno."

Parents take great care when choosing names for their children. Sometimes they name them after their favorite relatives or even Bible characters. (Of course, there are plenty of names in the Bible they do NOT choose, such as Abishag, Elishama, Jaazaniah and Habazziniah.)

One of the methods parents use to encourage proper behavior in their children is reminding them that no matter where they are or what they are doing, they should always "remember who they are" and live up to their names. Parents want their children's choices and actions to be a reflection of the values they cherish bringing honor to the family name. Socrates once wrote: "Regard your name as the richest jewel you can possibly possess."

The word "Christian" includes the name of "Christ." When we claim the title of "Christian" as our own, it is imperative that we "remember who we are." Everything we do should bring honor to that name. Our bodies are a gift from God and the way we treat them is a reflection of how much we appreciate that gift. When we were children, we took our health for granted and were usually not concerned about eating nutritious foods in proper quantities. Given a choice, a child will generally choose junk over healthy food. But the Apostle Paul tells us, *"When I was a child, I spoke like a child, I thought like a child, I reasoned like a child; when I became an adult, I put an end to childish ways."* (1 Corinthians 13:11 - NRSV)

Not only are we called to put an end to childish ways, we are called to "remember who we are" and practice the verse in Colossians 3:17: *"Whatever you do, whether in word or deed, do it all in the name of the Lord Jesus, giving thanks to God the Father through him."*

> O Heavenly Father, breathe into our souls the love of whatsoever is true and beautiful and good. May we fear to be unfaithful, and have no other fear. Help us to remember that we are your children, and belong to you. ~ William Angus Knight (1836–1916)

**FOOD FOR THOUGHT**

~ Do I live up to the name of "Christian"?

~ Is there anything I do that God might consider childish?

~ In what way are my actions a true reflection of the values I cherish?

## CHOOSE LIFE

Life is full of decisions. When our grandson, Ben Edwards, was 21, he shared a true-life illustration of the decision making process:

> Today, I woke up and I didn't want to go running. I wanted to lie in bed because my bed was so comfortable and it was raining outside. I felt like I wouldn't have fun running, my muscles would just hurt and I'd be cold and wet. It would be miserable and not worth it. I could just wake up and make some hot chai tea and sit with a blanket in my bed. It would be so much easier and I wouldn't have to go through all the effort. But I got myself up, put in my contacts, got dressed and went out into the cold.
>
> I didn't want to be there at the start, but as I began to run, I warmed up. My cold legs didn't cramp and were comfortable. It was peaceful, relaxing even - being alone and just hearing the rain. It was nothing like I expected or felt it would be. When I got back I was drenched, but my once cold apartment that I woke up in felt warm and cozy.
>
> After a hot shower, I weighed myself and found I had lost a pound. Since I've been running in the mornings, I feel more awake. It's also helped me with staying awake in classes and just feeling more productive. I'm glad I went running even though I didn't want to!

To Ben, it would have felt better to curl up under a blanket, but because he made the choice to run, he felt more alive. The Bible verse below tells us that we have choices to make and if we want the blessings, we must "choose life."

*"This day I call heaven and earth as witnesses against you that I have set before you life and death, blessings and curses. Now choose life, so that you and your children may live and that you*

*may love the LORD your God, listen to his voice and hold fast to him..."* (Deuteronomy 30:19-20a)

Life does not come with guarantees and many times there are no second chances. Each day we are bombarded with choices that can make the difference between a life filled with purpose and an aimless existence. I challenge you to go through one day and count how many choices you make that impact your health and your weight. I've heard that the number is well over 200. Those choices are not easy to make. There are always obstacles to overcome. Some are obvious, such as the cold and the rain. Some are hidden in our subconscious and stem from our background or previous experiences. But each can be overcome with God's help.

Making right choices has a snowball effect. When we do something good, we are happy with ourselves. Just as Ben said, "I'm glad I went running even though I didn't want to." Those positive emotions make it easier to make right choices the next time. When we "choose life," God never runs out of blessings!

> O God, by whom the meek are guided in judgment, and light rises up in darkness for the godly: Grant us, in all our doubts and uncertainties, the grace to ask what you would have us to do, that the Spirit of wisdom may save us from all false choices, and that in your light we may see light, and in your straight path may not stumble; through Jesus Christ our Lord.
> ~ Book of Common Prayer

**FOOD FOR THOUGHT**

~ Do I pray about my choices before I make them?

~ When is the last time I made a choice I regretted?

~ When I "choose life," what blessings await me?

# ITCHING TO BE STITCHING

My friend, Becki Flood, came for a visit from Oklahoma. We wanted her to have a good time and since she is a quilter, my husband and I took Becki and her daughter, Lesly, to tour the National Quilt Museum in Paducah, Kentucky. The museum attracts about 40,000 visitors annually and contains over 150 antique and contemporary quilts. I have never done any quilting, so I was thoroughly prepared for a long, boring afternoon. I found myself, however, blown away by the intricate craftsmanship, amazing creativity and sheer beauty of the quilts on display.

At this very moment, there is probably a multitude of quilters working diligently to create unique quilts for friends and loved ones. Hours of planning and labor go into creating just the perfect gift to represent a special bond of love.

One thing common to all quilters - they are always "itching to be stitching." They love what they do. Quilters get a bigger thrill out of shopping for material than for new clothes. They have even been known to visit fabric stores while on vacation. Even more important than loving what they do, however, is loving each other. There seems to be an instant camaraderie amongst quilters worldwide.

A master quilter can create a thing of beauty from an ordinary pile of scraps. To a quilter, a bed without a quilt is like a sky without stars. One of the crucial aspects of quilting is choosing the right fabric: the right texture, the right colors, the right patterns and even the right personality to fit the uniqueness of the person who will receive it.

To ensure the quilt will be cherished for years to come and then passed on to future generations, the craftsmanship must be superior. A serious quilter must have the gifts of patience, perseverance and tenacity. My talented friend, Sharon Johnson, has those gifts. One of my favorite quilts that she made has several types of birds on it. Because I have a new appreciation for quilts and because I am a bird lover, it combines the best of both worlds.

Our lives are like quilts. Sometimes life hands us only a pile of scraps, but it's up to us to use our God-given talents and creativity to make a masterpiece. Quilts often tell stories by reflecting memories or historical events. Our lives tell stories as well. What we value most in life is clearly demonstrated by our daily attitudes and actions.

Each piece of our life's quilt should reflect the fruit of the Spirit from Galatians 5:22-23: *"...the fruit of the Spirit is love, joy, peace, patience, kindness, goodness, faithfulness, gentleness and self-control..."* Because we have the support of the Holy Spirit, we should be "itching to be stitching" a life that is pleasing to our Heavenly Father and one that will inspire others in future generations.

> Lord, I pray that out of your glorious riches you may strengthen me with power through your Spirit in my inner being, so that you may dwell in my heart through faith. And I pray that, being rooted and established in love, I may have power, together with all the saints, to grasp how wide and long and high and deep is your love so that I may be filled to the measure of all your fullness.
> ~ based on Ephesians 3:16-19

**FOOD FOR THOUGHT**

~ What talents has God given me?

~ Am I doing anything creative with the "pile of scraps" life has handed me?

~ What would help me visualize the masterpiece God has in mind?

## WHEN GOD SAYS GO

I'm not sure about you, but I don't like bugs! Insects are not on my list of favorite things. There is one exception. I love butterflies. They have become the subject of many songs and poems throughout the years. Below is a stanza of a poem I wrote called, "The Butterfly."

> It looked like a bit of sunshine, dancing in the breeze.
> Darting in and among the flowers, it fluttered by with ease.
> Entranced by this tiny miracle, suddenly I knew!
> That God in all His mercy would gently guide me through.

We enjoy butterflies because they do not sting or become pests in our homes. It is considered good fortune if a butterfly lands on someone. An old Irish Blessing says, "May the wings of the butterfly kiss the sun and find your shoulder to light on."

Butterflies are brightly colored and fun to watch. They make the world a prettier place. There are about 24,000 known butterfly species throughout the world, ranging in size from $1/8^{th}$ inch to almost 12 inches. The name "butterfly" was created to describe the Yellow Brimstone butterfly in Europe. It was actually known as the butter-colored fly and later received the name butterfly.

It is one of nature's greatest mysteries how some butterflies are able to migrate long distances. Monarch butterflies flutter 2500 miles to Mexico each year. They all arrive at about the same time on the mountain peaks in an area that is only 60 square miles. A butterfly weighs about the same as two rose petals and only flies 12 miles per hour. To accomplish such a journey is amazing. How does something so small end up exactly where God wants it to be? Perhaps it is because a butterfly is obedient to its instincts. When God whispers, "Go," it does not procrastinate! For us to go the full distance God has planned, we do not have the luxury of procrastination. Butterflies don't contemplate the difficulty of their journey. If they did, they might be too discouraged to even try. They just go where God leads them.

In our struggles to maintain a healthy life style, we usually know what God wants us to do and where God wants us to go. Just like the Monarch butterfly, we have a long distance ahead of us, but if we listen, God is there to guide us. Isaiah 30:21 tells us: *"Whether you turn to the right or to the left, your ears will hear a voice behind you, saying, 'This is the way; walk in it.'"*

Ours is a spiritual journey of the utmost importance, but we do not have to worry about getting lost. Jesus simply said, *"Come, follow me…"* (Matthew 4:19) We never have to go anywhere that He has not already been.

When does God want us to begin our journey? NOW would be an excellent choice! Just like butterflies, we can navigate through life fulfilling His purpose for our lives, even if our "faith" weighs no more than two rose petals. Are we ready to go when God says, "Go"?

> O LORD, hear my prayer, listen to my cry for mercy; in your faithfulness and righteousness come to my relief. Let the morning bring me word of your unfailing love, for I have put my trust in you. Show me the way I should go, for to you I lift up my soul. Teach me to do your will, for you are my God; may your good Spirit lead me on level ground.   ~ Psalm 143:1,8,10

**FOOD FOR THOUGHT**

~ Am I ready to "go" when God says "go"?

~ How do I switch my focus from the difficulties of the journey to the blessings of the finish line?

~ What are some things that keep me from hearing God's voice?

# GOING BATTY

My husband went into the garage at our home in southern Illinois and picked up what he thought was a dried-up leaf on the floor. When it started to wiggle, he realized he was holding the wing of a small bat. He placed it on top of a bush outside and hoped it would survive.

Another "batty" experience occurred in West Virginia. We heard scratching noises from inside the downspout on the side of our garage. Thinking a bird was stuck inside the pipe, my husband put the water hose in the top and turned the water on. What flushed out the bottom of the pipe was a very angry bat with its teeth bared! My husband quickly covered the bat with a broom and swept it down the hill while I quickly went inside the house.

There are approximately 1000 species of bats in the world. They have been around since the age of the dinosaur. Most people do not like bats, but bats are very beneficial. They help get rid of mosquitos and keep gardens free of insects. One little brown bat can catch over 600 mosquitoes in an hour. A bat can consume almost 50% of its body weight in insects (moths, mosquitoes, flies and beetles) in one night. Another intriguing characteristic of bats is their unique sonar system. They are capable of emitting high-pitched squeals, up to 200 pulses per second. When the sound hits something, an echo bounces back to the bat's ears revealing specific details about the distance, size and shape of the object. This enables bats to fly safely in total darkness.

Sometimes life can drive us "batty." In an instant, our world can turn dark and dismal, making us feel like we are inside a pipe, scratching frantically to be free. Multiple misfortunes accumulate until we find ourselves angry enough to bare our teeth. During those stressful moments, we sometimes relax our goals of healthy eating. It seems to be the least of our worries. The more stress we experience, however, the more imperative it is to keep ourselves healthy. The foods we typically reach for when we are stressed are the ones that create further stress. They are usually high in caffeine, sugar, salt or fat. Consumption of the right nutrients is needed for energy, mental concentration and emotional stability.

Our greatest need in the midst of high stress is a spiritual one. A close relationship with the Almighty God of the Universe will soothe our fears even when our inner turmoil leaves every nerve ending raw. God is the great Comforter! *"Come to me, all you who are weary and burdened, and I will give you rest. Take my yoke upon you and learn from me, for I am gentle and humble in heart, and you will find rest for your souls."* (Matthew 11:28-29)

If we stay grounded in the God's Word, using the sonar system of the Holy Spirit to help us navigate through life's dark and frightening pathways, we will never go "batty" because *"...the Spirit helps us in our weakness. We do not know what we ought to pray for, but the Spirit himself intercedes for us..."* (Romans 8:26)

> O God and Father of us all, breathe upon us now your hallowed calm; lift the burden from our hearts, soothe the anxieties of our minds and send peace into our souls. Help us now to stand while in the shelter of your shadowing wings, and to be still, to wait for the revelation of your will that shall make us calm and strong.
> ~ W. E. Orchard

## FOOD FOR THOUGHT

~ What's been driving me batty lately?

~ With which weakness do I most need the help of the Holy Spirit?

~ In what ways does keeping my body healthy affect the way I handle stress?

# FIRST IMPULSE

I love sugar-free Lifesaver peppermints. I am also a creature of habit, so every night after I get into bed, I open the sliding wooden door in our bookcase headboard and take a peppermint from a container. I enjoy the pepperminty taste before I doze off to sleep. One night, my husband played a prank on me. When I reached my hand through the dark to get my mint, I discovered all the mints were stuck together. After struggling a bit, I finally turned on the light to see what the problem was. All the while my hubby was chuckling under his breath. He had used a sewing needle and thread to sew all the Lifesavers together. That was the first of a variety of "surprises" for me. On a different night, he replaced my entire supply with a supply of miniature super-balls. My husband's actions achieved one thing. My nightly peppermint treat was no longer a ritualistic habit driven by impulse.

We have a grandson who is driven by impulse also. David is a delightful child who enjoys life and has an action-oriented personality. If I have trouble getting anything to work, he wants to get his hands on it to try it for himself because he is sure he has the answer. He also does not believe in wasting unnecessary effort. If he walks into a room and doesn't know which light switch to use, he turns on all of them. It didn't take me long to discover that if David had been in a room, every light switch and ceiling fan would be on. Our dining room has a panel of four switches. That means, when David leaves the room, the light and ceiling fan are on in the dining room, and also in the adjacent Florida room.

One day, I finally told him to go through the house and figure out which light switch was the correct one to use so that the next time he went in a room, he would be able to turn on just the light he needed. And then, of course, turn it off when he left the room.

Many of us are guilty of being impulsive also, especially when it comes to eating. We do not take time to think before we put something into our mouths. The Bible has another word to describe impulsive behavior. It's called foolish. *"The fear of the LORD is the beginning of knowledge, but fools despise wisdom and discipline."* (Proverbs 1:7)

Impulsive eating, in the absence of wisdom, includes eating by the clock when we're not hungry, consuming everything on our plate just because it's there, eating to avoid hurting the cook's feelings, using food to soothe emotional stress and, most obviously, eating while watching television with no idea of quality or quantity.

When we find ourselves reacting instead of acting, perhaps our "first impulse" should be to pray for wisdom.

> Our Father God, we come to you as foolish children - children who try to live against your ways and end only in hurting ourselves. Forgive us. And give us sense - just plain sense - so we may see that your laws are your love, and that your laws are our life.
> ~ E. Stanley Jones (1884–1973)

## FOOD FOR THOUGHT

~ Do I tend to be impulsive or foolish or both?

~ How do I avoid hurting the cook's feelings when I'm not hungry?

~ When I really am hungry, do I throw all my taste bud switches "on" at once without thinking about what I really want?

# UNCONDITIONAL LOVE

My daughter Rhonda, who is a nurse, told me about her new patient. She said: "I'm dialyzing a prisoner tomorrow. Liver failure, hepatitis, kidney failure - comes with a guard."

That same week, I also learned our son, David, who had been out of prison for only three months, was again in trouble with the law. He first came to live with us in 1971 when he was 11. Since then, he has spent the majority of his life behind bars. My expectation, hope and desire was that by now, we would have realized his current direction was not taking him where he needed to be. I love him with all my heart, but sometimes feel angry with him for wasting his life when he could have accomplished so much.

Because our society has a tendency to be less than sympathetic to people when their problems are the direct results of their bad choices. I wondered how my daughter felt about doing dialysis on a prisoner, so I asked her if she was uncomfortable. Her response was…

> No it doesn't make me uncomfortable and I kind of have a heart for them. This guy today was in a lot of pain but can't have narcotics for pain. He was also quite incoherent from end stage liver failure induced encephalopathy. His brain is failing. He's only 43 and is bright yellow from jaundice. He was a DNR (do not resuscitate) but it was reversed until they could find family members to support the decision. They haven't found any.

I have always been impressed with the depth of Rhonda's compassion. Her response raised questions in my own mind. If I had been exposed to the same experiences and circumstances as this prisoner had been, would I have made the same wrong turns? They could not find any family members. How does it feel to have no family or at least none that care? What experiences shaped his sense of self-worth as a child? Did he feel loved?

What is God's attitude toward us when we do wrong? Many times our physical, emotional and spiritual problems are the direct result of our own choices. We feel guilty and envision His condemnation and anger, but if we repent, God is always ready to forgive. Psalm 116:5 tells us: *"The Lord is gracious and righteous; our God is full of compassion."*

Yes, sometimes I am angry with our son, David, but there is nothing I would not do for him. If we, as humans, can manage to show compassion to each other, imagine how much more our compassionate God can help us! I love the image in Hosea 11:4. *"I led them with cords of human kindness, with ties of love; I lifted the yoke from their neck and bent down to feed them."* Our Holy God is so full of love for His children that that he bends down to fulfill their needs!

God's love is unconditional! It is so vast and so deep, even when we cause our own problems through our choices, it's doubtful we will ever fully comprehend His love during our short time on earth.

> I will praise you, O Lord, among the nations; I will sing of you among the peoples. For great is your love, reaching to the heavens; your faithfulness reaches to the skies. Be exalted, O God, above the heavens; let your glory be over all the earth. ~ Psalm 57:9-11

**FOOD FOR THOUGHT**

~ How much compassion do I have for those who do not live up to my standards?

~ Do I allow guilt feelings to fester or do I take them immediately to the foot of the cross?

~ If I fully understood the depths of God's love, would it increase my desire to please Him?

# SLOW FADE

I had not seen Jane Cochram, my sister-in-Christ, for many years. She moved to Arizona, so we kept in touch though email and Christmas letters. I have always been able to tell her anything and not worry about her misunderstanding. She always seems to be in tune with my heart. Those are the best kind of friends.

I sent her an email that said, "Help! Your face is fading!" The *real* problem, of course, was not her face but my memory. I was trying to remember all of her facial features and my brain would not cooperate, so I asked her to send me a picture, which she did. The photo reminded me of how beautiful she is, inside and out.

I needed a "fresh look" at my friend because I had not recently been in close contact with her. Jesus offers us the opportunity to be in close contact with Him through prayer; so close that we can know His heart and know His will for our lives. We can know what pleases Him most. In 2 Peter 1:3,4, God even promised us that we may participate in His divine nature!

*"His divine power has given us everything we need for life and godliness through our knowledge of him who called us by his own glory and goodness. Through these he has given us his very great and precious promises, so that through them you may participate in the divine nature and escape the corruption in the world caused by evil desires."* (2 Peter 1:3,4)

When I was a small child, my mother was upset that I was spending a lot of time with one particular friend. She told me emphatically, "You are not allowed to play with her anymore. When you spend a lot of time with her, you act just like she does and I don't like the way she acts!" My mother wanted me to spend time with friends of good character so that some of their behavior would rub off on me. Wouldn't it be wonderful if we spent so much time with Jesus that His good character rubbed off on us?

People need a connection with God like plants need a connection to roots. It does not take long for flowers to begin to droop and fade after they have been cut. When flowers are no longer connected to their source of nourishment, they wither and die. When we cater to our own self-interests and ignore our Heavenly Father, His face begins to fade and with it goes our opportunity to *"participate in the divine nature and escape the corruption in the world caused by evil desires."* That lost opportunity leaves us at the mercy of our circumstances with no power to live above the temptations of this evil world.

There's a spiritual song by Casting Crowns called "Slow Fade." Fading is always gradual - so gradual that it sometimes goes unnoticed. Perhaps it's time for a fresh encounter with the living God to prevent the "slow fade"!

---

Christ be with me, Christ within me, Christ behind me,
Christ before me, Christ beside me, Christ to win me,
Christ to comfort and restore me.
Christ beneath me, Christ above me,
Christ in quiet, Christ in danger,
Christ in hearts of all that love me,
Christ in mouth of friend and stranger.
~ St. Patrick's Breastplate

---

## FOOD FOR THOUGHT

~ When was the last time I had a fresh encounter with God?

~ How much time do I spend with Jesus?

~ Do I consider my relationship with God vibrant? Why or why not?

## ODORIFEROUS

What's that smell? Anytime we detect a bad odor, we do not hesitate to complain. We don't like bad smells. That's probably why we wear deodorant and stay away from skunks. Yet there are thousands that gravitate to a stinky festival every spring - the Ramp Festival in Richwood, West Virginia. Ramps are wild plants, members of the onion family and supposedly the sweetest tasting and vilest smelling vegetables in nature. The odor is so objectionable that school children with ramp odor have been excused from school for several days.

We tasted ramps one time when we lived in Tornado, West Virginia. Once was enough! Ramps grow wild, are a staple for the locals and considered to have properties like a spring tonic. Members of the fire department start digging ramps a week before the festival and fill 20 - 30 trash bags with them. The festival has been attended by many famous people including: Harry Truman, Tennessee Ernie Ford, Eddie Arnold, Minnie Pearl and Dinah Shore.

One of the highlights of the festival is a recipe contest, which includes such delicacies as ramp candy, ramp cornbread, ramp au gratin and creamy ramp risotto (made from ramps, leeks, garlic, radicchio and Parmesan). One year the winner won the $500 top prize with his "ramped-up steak sandwich" and also walked off with the "most repugnant" award. He was given a basket full of breath mints and a bottle of Listerine.

There is an abundance of smelly things in this world we prefer to avoid – like doggy breath and rotten eggs for example. There is, however, an abundance of rich wonderful smells. I love the smell of the air after a spring thunderstorm, the sweet smell of a rose or the tantalizing odor of freshly-baked bread. My daughter, Rhonda, told me one day that she had baked bread with my granddaughter:

Christine and I made whole-wheat bread today in the bread machine. The bread's been in the machine for almost five hours and is almost done. It smells pretty good and Christine keeps coming in to look at it. She said, "I just can't get that bread off my mind!"

God considers us to be the sweet fragrance of Christ. *"For we are to God the aroma of Christ among those who are being saved and those who are perishing."* (2 Corinthians 2:15) There is no higher compliment than that. IF we are to be the "aroma of Christ," we must be more like Him in *everything* - not just when we are at church or when we get together with Christian friends. Our goal is to be like Jesus in our daily choices, our habits, our character and our love for others.

Probably most of us have never heard of ramps nor is visiting a Ramp Festival high on our list of priorities. We may prefer to steer clear of something as *odoriferous* as ramps. When it comes to *good* smells, however, it should be a high priority for us to be the "aroma of Christ" to the world! Hopefully, once they get to know us, they will say, "I just can't get Jesus off my mind!"

> O Lord my God, may I put off my old self, which is being corrupted by its deceitful desires, to be made new in the attitude of my mind and to put on the new self, created to be like you in true righteousness and holiness. ~ based on Ephesians 4:22-24

## FOOD FOR THOUGHT

~ How am I like Jesus in my daily choices?

~ Do I represent the sweet fragrance of Christ to my family?

~ How can I be the aroma of Christ to the world?

# THE STORMS OF LIFE

Have you ever noticed how the storms of life have a way of encouraging us to reevaluate our priorities? In 2009, our town of Marion, Illinois had what the media called an "inland hurricane." The 88 m.p.h. straight-line winds whipped through five counties with wind gusts up to 106 m.p.h. The Governor declared all five counties disaster areas.

Although our house escaped damage, we watched as the wind ripped tiles off our neighbor's roof and sailed them through the air like a deck of cards. Large, beautiful oak trees, all over town, were uprooted as easily as if they were spindly saplings. We lost our electricity for a period of 47 hours and some areas took as long as two weeks before power was restored.

When we lost electricity, I first worried about how I would finish my computer project. Then I fretted that we would not be able to watch the 6:00 p.m. news or take hot showers. As time went on, we thought about the food that would spoil in our freezer. When we realized the stores were not open, we wondered how we would be able to purchase necessities or put gasoline in our car. Neither telephones nor cell phones were working, so we were unable to monitor the safety of family and friends. My daughter and family live a half of a mile from us. What we thought was a simple solution (drive over to their house and check on them) turned out to be an impossible task because most side roads were blocked with large fallen trees.

Then we began to wonder about the hospitals and if the nurses could get to work. Were the neighborhood shut-ins safe in the dark? Would there be any house fires set by the careless use of candles? Was anyone hurt in the storm? Our initial reactions were focused on the comforts of life we were missing, but after a while, our reactions were focused on the needs of others. Compassion blossomed throughout town as volunteers pooled their talents, donating hours of labor to assist where needed. Members of the Southern Baptist Convention Disaster Relief Chainsaw Gang cut trees that were blocking the entrances to people's homes.

When the "storms of life" subside - the winds die down, the electricity comes back on and we get a hot cup of coffee and a hot shower - do we revert back to our old self-focused ways of thinking? How important are the thoughts and priorities that swirl in our heads in light of God's plans and purposes? How many of our daily activities are so securely wrapped in our own desires that they exclude everyone else, including God?

Maybe one purpose for the "storms of life" is simply to remind us that life is not all about us. The Bible tells us: *"Let no one seek his own, but each one the other's well-being."* (1 Corinthians 10:24)

---

Be, O God, a Refuge from the storm, and a Shadow from the heat. Even while we are lying safely in your arms, we are sometimes foolishly timid. Lo, help our unbelief, and, in your tenderness, assure us of your protection. You can make all things work together for good to them that love you. Let not calamity injure our souls; let not sorrow corrode our hearts.
~ John Hunter's Devotional Services (1892)

---

**FOOD FOR THOUGHT**

~ When things are going well, do I become more self-focused?

~ How do the storms of life help me to change my priorities?

~ What can I do to become more focused on others?

# FAMOUS LAST KICK

Our grandson, Brad, has always done well in sports, specifically soccer and track. In his freshman year of high school, he competed in the 1600m race. His father (our son, Bruce) relays the following information about a particular event:

> In the 1600m run, Brad was really seeking to break the five minute mark for the first time. He came close again last night with another personal best of five minutes, 6.3 seconds. There was a field of about 15 runners. Right from the start, Brad jumped out to the lead, but halfway through the second lap, he let two runners go ahead, but kept them at his front door. In the fourth and final lap, one of the leaders tuckered out and Brad blew by him. Then at the 150m mark, Brad pulled out his "famous last kick" and took the front runner with about 10 meters to go before the finish. Everyone was on their feet cheering. It was great!

These are the words of one proud papa. Obviously, Bruce had reason to be proud. When all of Brad's energy was gone, he was still able to reach down deep inside of himself and find the hidden resources necessary to excel.

The opposite was true of King Jeroboam of Jerusalem in Bible times. Jerusalem was a holy city; the ark of the Covenant was there. It was the center of worship for the Israelites, but instead of having the people journey all the way to Jerusalem, King Jeroboam set up substitute places of worship at Bethel and Dan in order to lessen their traveling. "*After seeking advice, the king made two golden calves. He said to the people, 'It is too much for you to go up to Jerusalem. Here are your gods, O Israel, who brought you up out of Egypt.' One he set up in Bethel, and the other in Dan.*" (1 Kings 12:28-29)

Is there a Bethel or a Dan in our lives as well? Perhaps it's that place that is easy to get to by following the path of least resistance. We want everything to be easy, including our prayer life. Just give us a formula that works every time - show us the right position, the right words to say and presto, God will reach down His finger of blessing to give us the answer we want.

We also want obtaining good physical health to be easy. Maybe if we eat the right amount of protein and drink enough water, we can still eat three brownies for dessert. Perhaps they will eventually develop a pill that will give us strong muscles with or without having to exercise. We are sometimes unwilling to reach down deep inside of us and draw on the hidden resources of God's power for that "famous last kick" that propels us to victory.

There are many times in life when we think we have gone as far as we can go. Our energy is gone, our spirit is spent and we end up living far below our capabilities. But we are able to do much more than we think we can. God's power is available! *"Oh, the utter extravagance of his work in us who trust him - endless energy, boundless strength!"* (Ephesians 1:19 - MSG) I think King David said it best in 2 Samuel 22:30: *"...with my God I can scale a wall."*

> Teach us, good Lord, to serve you as you deserve: to give, and not to count the cost; to fight, and not to heed the wounds; to toil, and not to seek for rest; to labor, and not to ask for any reward, except that of knowing that we do your holy will; through Jesus Christ our Lord. ~ Ignatius Loyola (1491-1556)

## FOOD FOR THOUGHT

~ Do I have any hidden resources I do not use?

~ Where or what is my Bethel or Dan?

~ Is my "last kick" famous?

# LEAVING A LEGACY

My mother, Esther, passed away in January of 2009 when she was 100 years old. God instructs us to learn from previous generations: *"This is what the Lord says: 'Stand at the crossroads and look; ask for the ancient paths, ask where the good way is, and walk in it, and you will find rest for your souls...'"* (Jeremiah 6:16) It's easy to learn from my mother's life because she left such a great legacy - not only through her stories, poems and piano music, but also through her generous, unselfish nature to anyone in need. Her life blessed almost everyone she met.

Unwittingly or not, we all leave legacies for future generations. The question is what kind of legacy are we leaving? If we were asked to write what our headstones would read, I wonder what we would choose. Most of us prefer not to think that far ahead and therefore would be challenged by the assignment. Everything we say and do and believe is written daily in the hearts of those who know us.

When our granddaughter, Meghan, was 11 years old, she had a school assignment to write poetry and to make a list of her favorite poems by other poets. She said:

>  I had fun writing the poems for my poem book. I enjoyed reading my grandma's and my nana's poems. I learned it was not so hard to write a poem and it was fun to read it when it was all done. My favorite poems are 'Time Passes On' and 'One Night I Dreamt of Heaven' written by my nana.
>
>  When my nana died, my brother and I read these poems my nana wrote. They were interesting and talked of God's love and promises for us. I will always remember these two poems because it was an honor to read them at her funeral, and I will always remember my Nana.

Meghan was especially brave to have read poetry at the funeral of someone she loved. My mother had no idea of the impact she had on her children, her grandchildren and her great-grandchildren, as well as friends and neighbors. Although, in her humble mind, she was just trying to live her life as best she could, her life and the choices she made left a legacy for all of us.

What kind of legacy are we leaving? Realizing that our influence - good or bad - will live for years to come may inspire us to take notice of the trail we are leaving. The legacy my mother left was one of a life lived from the heart. She advises us to do the same in the first stanza of her poem, "Time Passes On."

> Time passes on and what does it bring?
> Time brings changes to everything.
> How do you cope? Where do you start?
> The best thing to do is follow your heart!

The heart is made for love - not love of self, but love for God and others. Following our hearts means listening to the still, small voice of God and making the daily choices that leave an inspiring trail for others to follow. That, my friends, is the best legacy of all!

---

Breathe in me, O Holy Spirit, that my thoughts may all be holy. Act in me, O Holy Spirit, that my work, too, may be holy. Draw my heart, O Holy Spirit, that I love but what is holy. Strengthen me, O Holy Spirit, to defend all that is holy. Guard me, then, O Holy Spirit, that I always may be holy. ~ St. Augustine (354-430)

---

**FOOD FOR THOUGHT**

~ What can I learn from previous generations?

~ How much responsibility to I feel for future generations?

~ If I could choose one of my traits to pass on to my children, which one would it be?

## DREAM ON

What is your dream? Do you remember what you dreamt when you were young? Maybe, as you gazed into the stars, you could see yourself flying through the sky. Maybe before Christmas, you saw yourself receiving a shiny red bicycle. As you grew older, your thoughts were probably filled with finding just the right person to marry. Then you thought about owning a home. It's exciting to open up our imaginations and explore all the possibilities! Many times, however, our dreams evaporate as quickly as a drop of water on a hot skillet.

My daughter, Kerry, has a friend named Mary Aslyer. One time Mary shared her dream with me. At the time she was living in a trailer home with her husband and three small children, but dreamt of the day she could move her family into a real house. Listen to the way she describes her dream. It is so vivid and real we have x-ray vision into her very heart and soul:

> My dream is a house of my own; something big and rambling with a huge yard. My bedroom will be filled with windows…drenched every morning with soft shafts of sunlight. My kitchen will be bright and cheerful…smelling of freshly baked bread. My family room will be constantly messy, strewn with toys and filled with signs of life and love. My dining room will not be a showpiece, but rather the center of our life.
>
> I'll have a huge old oak table lovingly restored to its former glory - the kind of table you wish could talk so it could share the secrets it has heard over the years - stories of jubilance, sorrow, puppy love and dark nights of the soul. The centerpiece would be a huge white, slightly chipped crockery vase filled daily with fresh wildflowers gathered by my baby girl.
>
> In the yard will be an ancient tree. In its branches will be a tree house built by the boys and their dad. Another branch will

host a swing and carved in the tree trunk will be a heart and the initials of my daughter's first secret love. And last, but not least, will be my front porch. At one end, a wooden porch swing cradled beneath boughs of wisteria. Private, yet strategically placed, so when sitting in his recliner, Dad can discreetly view it through delicate lacy curtains. Yeah, this is my dream!

Can you see Mary's dream? Can you feel her desire? Mary ended up achieving her ambitions and so can we. What is your dream? Do you long for a healthy body? Do you long to be set free from the tyranny of self-destructive habits? Never give up! There are some things that will never materialize without a dream.

Dream on, regardless of the heartache of past failures. Dream on, regardless of how much water is already over the dam. Dream on, regardless of the giants looming on the horizon. God is the God of the "possible." Jesus said in Luke 18:27, *"What is impossible with men is possible with God."* Dream on!

---

O God of my body, I would have it at your best. You have made me for health and rhythm; help me to present this body of mine for you to make out of it the very finest instrument for your purposes. Help every brain cell and every tissue and every nerve to be the strings upon which your creative fingers shall play and bring out undreamed-of harmony and effectiveness.

~ E. Stanley Jones (1884–1973)

---

## FOOD FOR THOUGHT

~ What is my dream?

~ How have past failures dimmed my vision?

~ How much hope do I have for the future? What can I do to have more hope?

## CONCLUSION

Somewhere in these meditations, I pray there is one "just for you!" If you feel a renewed hope, we will give God the praise. If you feel inspired to make a change in your life, let me encourage you to seize the opportunity and take action now. In other words, "strike while the iron is hot."

If you feel a stirring of hope that change is possible, don't put it off until tomorrow or next week. Don't save it for a New Year's resolution. Don't wait until after all the freshly-baked cookies have been eaten. Don't delay until you have more time to plan your menus. Martin Luther said, "How soon not now becomes never!" Most of all, don't put it off because you are afraid of failure. Start now!

Start now and give it your best effort. The pianist and organist at our church (Judy Hopkins and Sharon Disney) both have an abundance of God-given talent. When they play on Sunday mornings, we are ushered directly into the presence of God. They did not achieve their abilities through wishful thinking, but instead by dedication and hard work. There is another element to their playing that can be clearly recognized: they believe in what they are doing. You can hear their passion in every note.

Let's apply these concepts to our new motivation for self-care. In addition to perseverance and determination, it will take passion and a burning desire to please and honor the One who created us.

Somewhere deep inside each of us is a passion for excellence. If we can generate a clear vision of the freedoms and blessings that await us, that passion will bubble to the surface and lead us to reach our goals.

## THE GOAL

The goal was lofty, the passion deep;
I was determined to win.
I could already see myself with the prize;
My face wore a confident grin.

Each day I scheduled my plan of attack,
Faithfully toiling away;
Proud of my progress, I relaxed my aim
And had ample time to play.

One morning I awoke and it seemed to me
That from the recesses of my mind,
A faint recollection struggled to emerge...
The prize for which long I had pined.

My lofty goal had faded from sight
Like a slowly dying ember;
I was further away than when I began
Because I forgot to remember.

~ *Idella Pearl Edwards*

The poem speaks of a "lofty goal." How much loftier can our goal be than to appreciate and care for the amazing bodies God created for us? A healthy body gives us more freedom to accomplish the things God calls us to do. That should be more than enough reason to let our passions run deep! That should be more than enough reason to shrink our bodies, grow our souls and refresh our spirits.

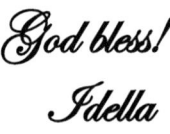

*God bless!*
*Idella*

## SCRIPTURES ON HOPE

Why are you downcast, O my soul? Why so disturbed within me? Put your hope in God, for I will yet praise him, my Savior and my God.
~ Psalm 43: 5

Blessed is he whose help is the God of Jacob, whose hope is in the LORD his God, the Maker of heaven and earth, the sea, and everything in them - the LORD, who remains faithful forever. ~ Psalm 146: 5-6

But blessed is the man who trusts in the LORD, whose confidence is in him. He will be like a tree planted by the water that sends out its roots by the stream. It does not fear when heat comes; its leaves are always green. It has no worries in a year of drought and never fails to bear fruit.
~ Jeremiah 17:7-8a

But as for me, I watch in hope for the LORD, I wait for God my Savior; my God will hear me. ~ Micah 7: 7

Oh! May the God of green hope fill you up with joy; fill you up with peace, so that your believing lives, filled with the life-giving energy of the Holy Spirit, will brim over with hope! ~ Romans 15: 13 (MSG)

I pray also that the eyes of your heart may be enlightened in order that you may know the hope to which he has called you, the riches of his glorious inheritance in the saints, and his incomparably great power for us who believe. ~ Ephesians 1: 18-19a

We have this hope as an anchor for the soul, firm and secure. It enters the inner sanctuary behind the curtain, where Jesus, who went before us, has entered on our behalf. ~ Hebrews 6: 19-20a

Let us hold unswervingly to the hope we profess, for he who promised is faithful. ~ Hebrews 10: 23

Therefore, prepare your minds for action; be self-controlled; set your hope fully on the grace to be given you when Jesus Christ is revealed.
~ 1 Peter 1:13

## TEMPTED

Lord, we are tempted, more often than not
To take the easy way out;
We are tempted to want more than our share,
We are tempted to fear and to doubt.

But, Lord, you have taught us in your Holy Word
That Satan is the father of lies;
If we seek the Truth, he cannot deceive us,
No matter how hard he tries.

Jesus, you have shown us by your example
That our life can be glorious;
And you have given us all we need
In order to be victorious!

~ *Idella Pearl Edwards*

## HOW GREAT?

How great would my life become, I wonder,
If I became healthy and trim,
If I left all the excess baggage behind
And discovered what it's like to be slim.

How great would my life become, I wonder,
(The best is yet to be seen)
If I exercised faithfully day after day
And became a lean machine.

How great would my life become, I wonder,
If my spiritual life were refined,
If I learned to love the Lord, my God,
With heart, soul, strength and mind.

~ *Idella Pearl Edwards*

# ACKNOWLEDGMENTS

Acknowledgment is gratefully expressed to the authors and publishers who have granted permission for use of quotations.

1. Beatrice Page, *The Bracelet,* (The Bobbs-Merrill Company, Inc., 1953), p. 14. Used by permission of Emily Page-Steacy.

2. Used by permission of Ruth Seamands.

3. Carole Lewis, *Stop It!,* (Regal Books From Gospel Light, Carole Lewis, 2005), p. 10. Used by permission of Carole Lewis.

4. E. Stanley Jones, *The Way,* (Abingdon-Cokesbury Press, 1946), p. 75. Used by permission of Eunice Jones Mathews.


I am deeply indebted to the following people for their time and effort in proofing various sections of my book and for their warm words of encouragement:

- Rhonda Andersen
- Judy Beard
- Rev. Ken Burgard
- Jack Edwards
- Jean Malone
- Kim Vanderhelm
- Tori Westrick

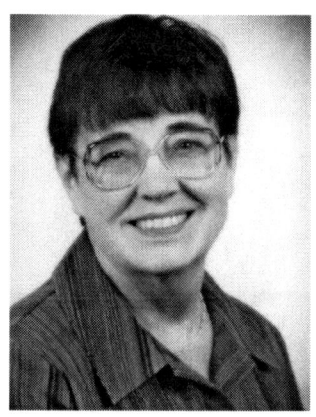

## ABOUT THE AUTHOR

Idella Edwards retired from the State of Oklahoma in 2005 but has lived in eight different states. She currently resides in Marion, Illinois where she is an active member of Aldersgate United Methodist Church, team-teaching an adult Sunday School class, singing in the choir, participating in United Methodist Women and leading a weight-loss group called Body & Soul. She is a published poet and newspaper columnist.

Born and raised in Aurora, Illinois, Idella attended Olivet Nazarene University and received a degree from College of DuPage. She and her husband, Jack, have five children and twelve grandchildren. They spent several years coordinating Lay Witness Missions and have been Certified Lay Speakers for the United Methodist Church since 1990.

Previous publications include "MAGNIFY, Inspirational Poetry for the Soul" and poetry published in various Christian magazines.

CPSIA information can be obtained at www.ICGtesting.com
Printed in the USA
LVOW080338260612

287526LV00005B/1/P

9 780615 653556